# Clinical Nuclear Medicine in Neurology

Andrea Varrone
Silvia Morbelli • Valentina Garibotto
Editors

# Clinical Nuclear Medicine in Neurology

## An Atlas of Challenging Cases

Springer

*Editors*
Andrea Varrone
Centre for Psychiatry Research
Department of Clinical Neuroscience
Karolinska Institutet and Stockholm
Health Care Services
Stockholm
Sweden

Silvia Morbelli
Nuclear Medicine Unit
IRCCS Ospedale Policlinico San
Martino
Genova
Italy

Valentina Garibotto
Geneva University and Geneva
University Hospitals
Geneva
Switzerland

ISBN 978-3-030-83597-2 ISBN 978-3-030-83598-9 (eBook)
https://doi.org/10.1007/978-3-030-83598-9



This Springer imprint is published by the registered company Springer Nature Switzerland AG
The registered company address is: Gewerbestrasse 11, 6330 Cham, Switzerland

# Preface

The applications of Nuclear Medicine in neurodegenerative disorders, epilepsy as well as in neuroimmunology and neuro-oncology have expanded in the last two decades. The main reason for such increase in the number of applications is the wide use of PET imaging with [$^{18}$F]FDG, with tracers targeting pathological processes such as amyloid and tau aggregates, as well as with [$^{18}$F]Fluorodopa, $^{68}$Ga-DOTATOC/DOTATATE, and [$^{18}$F] Fluoroethyltyrosine, using hybrid imaging with CT and MRI. Dopamine transporters (DAT) SPECT has also become a diagnostic imaging modality widely used in clinical practice.

Nowadays, challenges might derive from atypical or incomplete clinical presentations requiring combined interpretation of both functional and morphological images acquired with hybrid imaging as well as with stand-alone modalities. In particular, the expansion of hybrid imaging with the broad implementation of PET/MRI systems has contributed to a more integrated diagnostic approach in nuclear neurology, combining multimodal MR and PET imaging. These developments have improved the diagnostic work-up but have also contributed to more technical complexity. Similarly, nuclear medicine tools are increasingly integrated as biomarkers to improve accuracy of clinical diagnosis and to identify disease trajectories that characterise the natural history of neurological diseases. There is therefore a need for continuous education in Clinical Nuclear Medicine, as well as for updates of the procedures and software development that are necessary to achieve more objective reading and diagnostic interpretations of the brain scans.

The purpose of this book is to present a collection of challenging cases, in which the use of nuclear medicine examinations, in combination with MRI and optimised user-independent methods of image processing and analysis, interpreted in association with the clinical presentation and context, has contributed to the final diagnosis. The chapters describe cases of patients with neurodegenerative disorders, epilepsy and brain tumours as well as all less frequent clinical scenarios such as autoimmune encephalitis, Creutzfeldt-Jacob and Huntington's disease. In all cases clinical question, main findings and possible interpretations are highlighted. The added value of semi-quantification and voxel-based analysis and the need to compare metrics with normal subjects' database have been also discussed when appropriate. Finally, most relevant papers and guidelines are also provided as reference for the reader.

Our intention with this book was to provide guidance on the correct interpretation of nuclear medicine procedures for the diagnosis of neurological disorders and exemplify more and less common variants that may render the interpretation of nuclear medicine images complex.

A recurrent observation across cases is the importance of a thorough analysis of the clinical question, an in-depth knowledge of tracer behaviour and potential pitfalls, and a multidisciplinary synthesis of clinical, laboratory and imaging findings. The combination of all these elements is key for an accurate interpretation and required in order to fully exploit the great potential of nuclear medicine methods, reminding the importance for a training that emphasises not only the technical expertise but also the clinical expertise of nuclear medicine specialists.

We hope that these cases will support the clinical work of specialists and will serve as support for teaching new professionals. We thank all the contributing authors for their expertise and competence that made possible to realise this unique collection of challenging cases.

Stockholm, Sweden — Andrea Varrone
Genova, Italy — Silvia Morbelli
Geneva, Switzerland — Valentina Garibotto

# Contents

# Section I

# Nuclear Medicine Cases of Dementia and Movement Disorders

# Case 1: Mild Cognitive Impairment (MCI)—[18F]FDG and Amyloid PET

Silvia Morbelli and Alberto Miceli

## Background

Mild cognitive impairment (MCI) corresponds to a slight but measurable decline in cognitive abilities, including memory and thinking skills but still in absence of a noticeable impact of their activities of daily leaving. Patients with MCI are at an increased risk of developing Alzheimer's (AD) or other dementia. Several biomarkers are available to support the diagnosis of AD and other neurodegenerative diseases at the stage of MCI both in clinical and research settings. Even in absence of disease modifying drugs an early accurate diagnosis may allow to apply lifestyle changes or logistical arrangements before disability has developed. Moreover after an early diagnosis, patients can be included in clinical trials involving new potentially effecting experimental intervention. Considering imaging biomarkers, [$^{18}$F]fluorodeoxyglucose ([$^{18}$F]FDG) PET and amyloid PET imaging provide valuable and complementary information. As neurodegenerative diseases are associated with deposition of pathological proteins both in the brain and in peripheral organs, their classification is protein based. However, as the progressive dysfunction and loss of neurons leads to distinct involvement of functional systems, major clinical symptoms are mainly determined by the anatomical regions showing neuronal and synaptic dysfunction (which in turn do not necessarily reflect the molecular changes in the background). Neuropathological studies have demonstrated that in AD and in other neurodegenerative diseases synaptic degeneration precedes neuronal death for a substantial period of time. This phenomenon can be reflected by the in vivo FDG uptake that is strongly correlated to cerebral synaptic density and activity thus reflecting the presence of neurodegeneration (as originally described from the study by Magistretti and Pellerin see suggested readings). For this reason, the hypometabolic pattern highlighted by [$^{18}$F]-FDG PET provides information on the extent and localization of neuronal dysfunction, and thus on the endophenotype of neuronal injury. On the other side, amyloid PET allows noninvasive, in vivo detection of amyloid plaques, one of the main neuropathological landmarks of AD with high sensitivity and specificity. When comparing the ability to predict progression to Alzheimer's dementia, a slightly higher sensitivity has been reported for amyloid PET over [$^{18}$F]FDG PET, although [$^{18}$F]FDG PET has a higher specificity and a better accuracy for predicting shortterm progression (see Blazhenets et al. from the suggested reading for further

S. Morbelli (✉) · A. Miceli
IRCCS Ospedale Policlinico San Martino, Genoa, Italy

Nuclear Medicine Unit, Department of Health Sciences, University of Genoa, Genoa, Italy
e-mail: silviadaniela.morbelli@hsanmartino.it


A. Varrone et al. (eds.), *Clinical Nuclear Medicine in Neurology*,
https://doi.org/10.1007/978-3-030-83598-9_1

details). Following the definition provided by panel commissioned by the National Institute on Aging and the Alzheimer's Association (NIA-AA), guidelines to define preclinical AD have been established for research purposes. The NIA-AA criteria were based on a conceptual model of the pathophysiology of AD and on the timeframe in which AD biomarkers become positive. In this model amyloid biomarkers (PET amyloid imaging and cerebrospinal fluid (CSF) Aβ42) become abnormal first; then biomarkers of neuronal injury and degeneration (CSF tau, FDG PET, and anatomic MRI) become abnormal later thus more strictly reflecting time of onset and severity of clinical symptoms. In this framework, suspected non-AD pathophysiology (SNAP) is a biomarker-based concept denoting AD-like neurodegeneration in individuals without brain amyloidosis. The term SNAP was first described in 450 clinically normal individuals aged >70 years were classified using amyloid plaque density assessed by PET, brain metabolism assessed by [$^{18}$F]FDG PET and hippocampal volume assessed by MRI. 23% of participants had neurodegeneration without amyloidosis (Amyloid negative, Neurodegeneration positive). The term SNAP was used to convey the notion that the latter group did not represent preclinical AD, but rather had biomarker evidence of non-AD neurodegenerative processes. Accordingly, SNAP is a biomarker-based concept that allows the characterization of both cognitively normal and impaired individuals clinically matching the presence of AD but in absence of brain amyloidosis. In recent years several possible underlying etiologies have been recognized in patients classified as SNAP. Underlying etiologies include hippocampal sclerosis, TDP-43 pathology and primary age-related tauopathy (PART). The identification of SNAP patients and the evidence that MCI patients classified as SNAP have a greater risk of clinical or cognitive decline than amyloid and neurodegeneration MCI have implications for counseling patients with subjective cognitive complaints or MCI in clinical practice.

## Patient's Characteristics

### Woman, 76-Years-Old; Right-Handed; 13 Years of Education

At first evaluation she complained of gradually onset, immediate memory deficit for 1 year, that was confirmed by the husband. She was aware of the deficit which caused anxiety and an apparent, continuous 'state of confusion'. General medical and neurological examinations were inconclusive.

Blood and urine screening were normal. No major medical history No vascular risk factors. She was not on any medication. No significant depression (GDS 15 = 4).

Everyday functioning was essentially preserved because she used alternative strategies, such as writing in agenda what she has to do time by time. Instrumental (IADL) and Basic (BADL) Activities of Daily Living = all main functions preserved. The ApoE genotype: Ɛ2/3.

**Neuropsychological assessment:**

- MMSE = 27/30;
- *Executive functions*: normal (TMT A and B and Symbol digit and Stroop tests);
- *Memory tests*: Episodic memory (Babcock story) = borderline.
- Free and Cued Selective Reminding Test (Grober Buschke) = low values in immediate memory and delayed recall with borderline values after cueing.
- Corsi's spatial memory = normal.
- Digit span for working memory = normal.
- *Visuoconstruction* = normal (Constructional praxis and Clock test).
- *Language* = normal (phonological verbal fluency and semantic verbal fluency).

The patient was classified as a single-domain amnestic Mild Cognitive Impairment. An MRI scan was performed (Fig. 1).

Given the clinical presentation and MRI findings the patient was classified as suspected amnestic MCI due to AD. To further support this diagnosis a brain [$^{18}$F]FDG PET/CT was performed (Fig. 2).

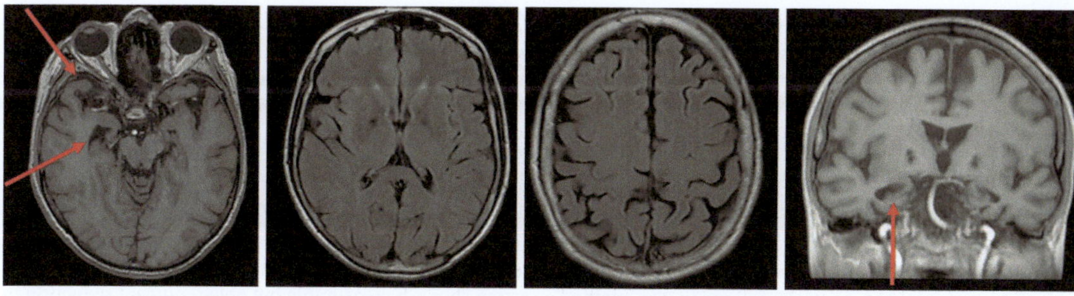

**Fig. 1** Axial T1-weighted MRI images and T2 in sagittal view showing significant atrophy of the right medial temporal lobe and moderate atrophy of the right temporal pole (red arrows). No significant parietal or posterior cingulate atrophy. No significant ventricular enlargement. Absence of vascular lesions

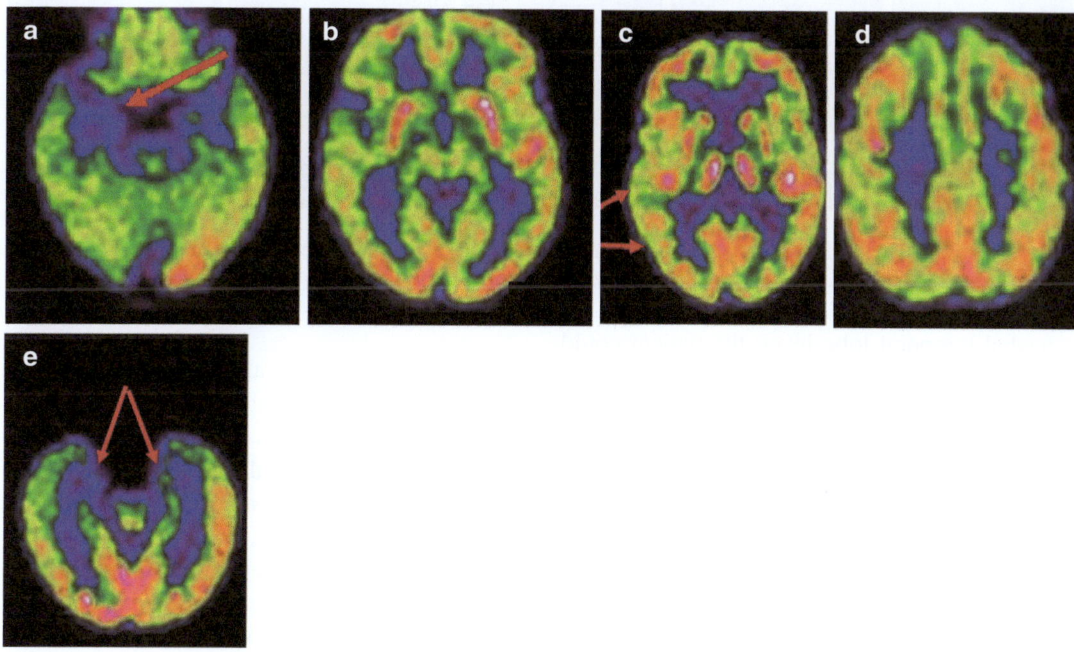

**Fig. 2** [$^{18}$F]FDG PET images oriented along the bicommissural line (**a**–**d**) and along the hippocampal axes (**e**) showing hypometabolism in the right medial temporal lobe (red arrows in **a** and **e**) and a mild asymmetry (right $<$ left) in temporal lateral cortex (**a** and **c**)

Given the results of the brain FDG PET scan (Figs. 2 and 3), imaging findings were largely insufficient to confirm MCI due to AD and the patients and a clinical and neuropsychological follow up was performed 1 year later. Neuropsychological assessment highlighted a similar profile with further worsening of cueing in delayed recall. In particular, episodic memory test was abnormal and the Free and Cued Selective Reminding Test showed low values in immediate memory and delayed recall with low values after cueing.

Given the increasing state of anxiety generated by the subjective insight of the cognitive deficit the patients was then submitted to an amyloid PET scan with $^{18}$F-Florbetaben (Fig. 4).

The patient falls into the 'Suspected non Alzheimer Pathology', SNAP, category. As mentioned SNAP is not a diagnosis. In this case, given the prominent and relative isolated atrophy

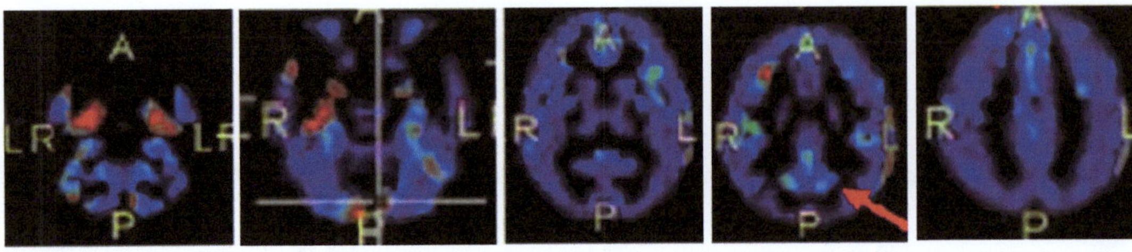


**Fig. 3** Results of whole brain voxel-wise analysis with respect to age-matched controls following the method described by Herholz et al. 2002 (cfr suggested readings). In red color clusters of significant hypometabolism with respect to controls in both medial temporal lobes. The red arrow shows a measurable but not significant reduction in precuneus/posterior cingulate metabolism with respect to controls

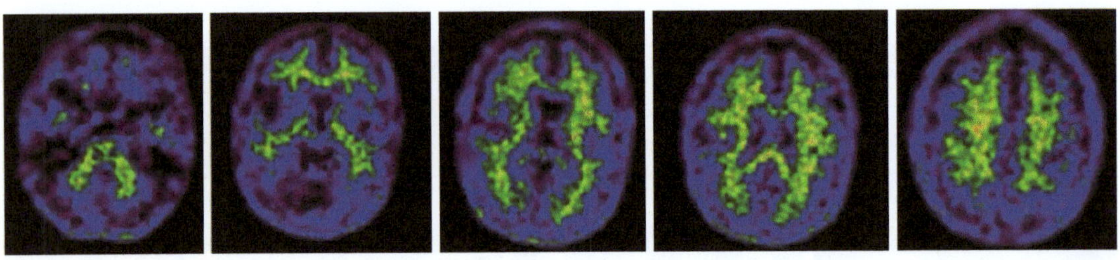

**Fig. 4** Negative amyloid PET scan. A preserved contrast is highlighted between the expected non-specific uptake in white matter and the uptake in the white matter. The gray matter uptake is always below the uptake in white matter

at medial temporal lobe level, the patient could be affected by hippocampal sclerosis or PART. The speed of progression of cognitive impairment as well as the lack of progression of measurable atrophy outside the medial temporal lobe might allow to further support this hypothesis overtime in this group of patients. This was indeed the case of the present patients at follow up (clinical stability and no significant progression of atrophy overtime).

**Teaching Points**

- SNAP is a label applied to patient (or healthy elderly subjects) undergoing neuroimaging biomarkers and proven to have AD-like neurodegeneration on MRI or FDG PET or both, but with a negative amyloidosis biomarkers.
- Demographics: SNAP subjects tend to be older than both A+N− subjects and AD patients.
- Genetics: the prevalence of ApoE epsilon 4 genotype (about 10%) is lower than in AD patients and even lower than in the general population.
- Neuropsychology: no distinct feature in SNAP as a whole, but impairment in other tests than Memory is milder than in amyloid-positive pts.; semantic verbal fluency is specifically preserved in patients with Hippocampal Sclerosis.
- Neuroradiology: Medial temporal lobe atrophy is often severe (both in PART and Hippocampal Sclerosis).
- Nuclear Medicine: FDG PET has overlap with AD but may show only minor changes.
- Progression: SNAP subjects progress to MCI or dementia more slowly and less frequently than patients A+N+ but more quickly than patients A−N−, and similarly as patients A+N.

## Suggested Reading

Blazhenets G, Ma Y, Sörensen A, et al. Predictive value of 18FFlorbetapir and 18FFDG PET for conversion from mild cognitive impairment to Alzheimer dementia. J Nucl Med. 2020;61:597–603.

Burnham SC, Bourgeat P, Doré V, Savage G, Brown B, Laws S, et al. Clinical and cognitive trajectories in cognitively healthy elderly individuals with suspected non-Alzheimer's disease pathophysiology (SNAP) or Alzheimer's disease pathology: a longitudinal study. Lancet Neurol. 2016;15:1044–53.

Dani M, Brooks DJ, Edison P. Suspected non-Alzheimer's pathology - is it non-Alzheimer's or non-amyloid? Ageing Res Rev. 2017;36:20–31.

Herholz K, Salmon E, Perani D, Baron JC, Holthoff V, Frölich L, et al. Discrimination between Alzheimer dementia and controls by automated analysis of multicenter FDG PET. Neuroimage. 2002;17:302–16.

Jack CR Jr, Bennett DA, Blennow K, Carrillo MC, Dunn B, Elliott C, et al. NIA-AA research framework: towards a biological definition of Alzheimer's disease. Alzheimers Dement. 2018;14:535–62.

Magistretti PJ, Pellerin L. Astrocytes couple synaptic activity to glucose utilization in the brain. News Physiol Sci. 1999;14:177–82.

# Case 2: Alzheimer's Disease—[$^{18}$F] FDG, Tau, and Amyloid PET

Javier Arbizu and Juan Fernando Bastidas

## Case Summary

A 64-year-old woman with postsecondary education and a previous history of depression, displayed loss of memory and repetitive behavior. She had difficulty remembering the names of people and objects, as well as recent conversations. Nevertheless, she was autonomous for the basic and elaborated activities of daily living, cooked without difficulties, had no problem cleaning and/or organizing the house and managed her money well. The neurological examination was normal, and the Mini Mental State Examination (MMSE) score was 25/30. The neuropsychological assessment revealed a multidomain mild cognitive impairment (MCI). On the other hand, she showed normal values for thyroid profile, vitamin B12, and folic acid.

J. Arbizu (✉) · J. F. Bastidas
Department of Nuclear Medicine, Clinica Universidad de Navarra, University of Navarra, Pamplona, Spain
e-mail: jarbizu@unav.es

## Images/Findings

A brain magnetic resonance imaging (MRI) scan showed a discrete cortical atrophy predominantly in the frontal and parietal lobes. Due to the atypical presentation and uncertain etiology of the MCI, she performed additional complementary examinations. Specifically, she carried out a brain positron emission tomography scan (PET) with [$^{18}$F]fluorodeoxiglucose (FDG-PET), and an amyloid PET scan using [$^{18}$F]Florbetaben (amyloid PET).

The FDG-PET showed a moderate hypometabolism in parieto-temporal association areas, particularly on the left side, and in the lateral region of the occipital cortex. Interestingly, there was no evidence of posterior cingulate involvement (Fig. 1). In the amyloid PET study, a pathological cortical increase in the uptake of the radiotracer was observed in the frontal, parietal, temporal, posterior cingulate, precuneus, as well as basal ganglia (Fig. 2), consistent with an increased density of cortical β-amyloid neuritic plaques. In the quantitative analysis, the average Standardized Uptake Value Ratio to cerebellum (SUVR) was 2.00 (normal ≤1.35 for Florbetaben-PET) [1].

According to these findings, the neurologist offered the patient to participate in a phase III clinical trial (monoclonal antibody against amyloid). In addition to the treatment opportunity, this trial brought the patient to conduct a tau-PET



A. Varrone et al. (eds.), *Clinical Nuclear Medicine in Neurology*,
https://doi.org/10.1007/978-3-030-83598-9_2

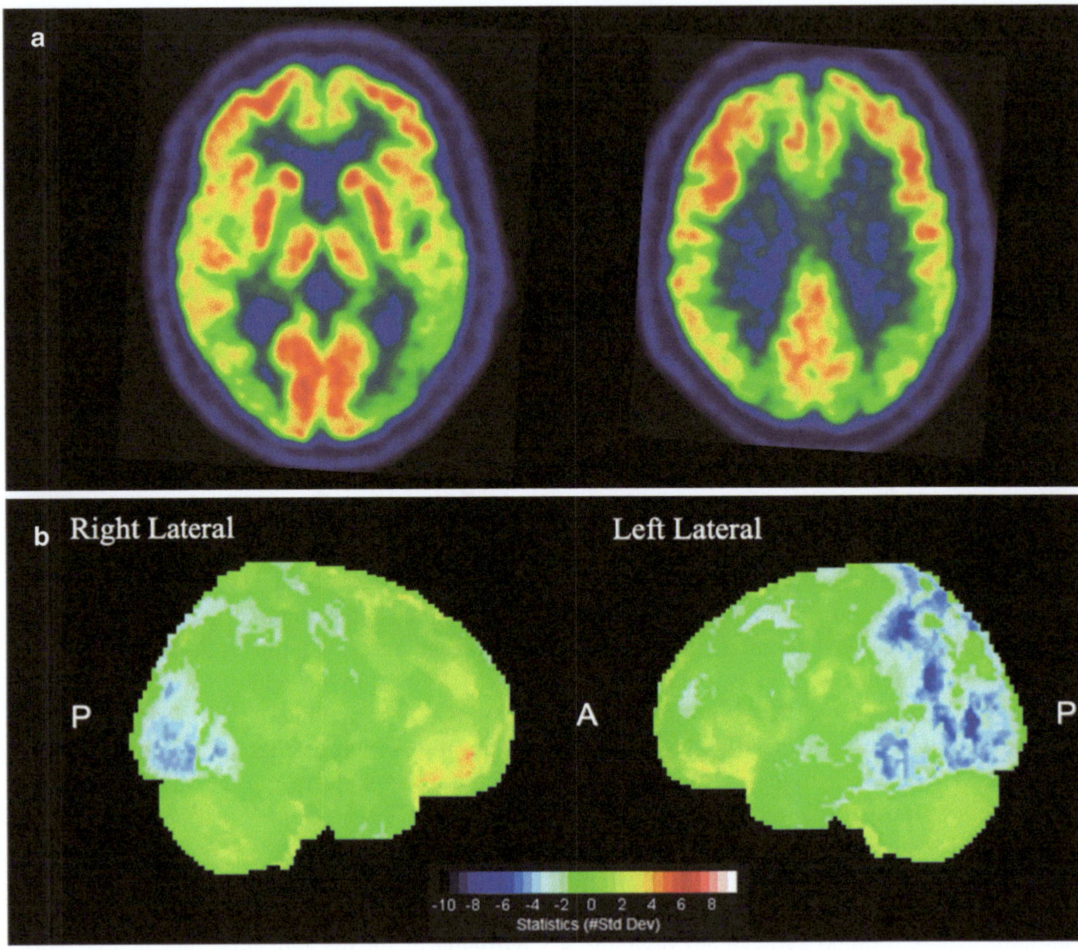


**Fig. 1** PET/CT with [$^{18}$F]FDG. (**a**) Sequential axial slices showing hypometabolism predominantly in left parieto-temporal region and the lateral region of the occipital cortex bilaterally. (**b**) Three-dimensional stereotactic surface projection (3D-SSP) maps (Syngo via database comparison, Siemens). Cortical areas with significant hypometabolism of FDG (>2 SD) are shown in blue

scan using [$^{18}$F]GTP1 (GTP1-PET). This study showed a high uptake in the lateral temporal, parietal and posterior cingulate cortex. Additionally, the study showed an increased tracer deposition in the lateral-occipital cortex bilaterally, which correlated with the clinical phenotype, specifically with the visual agnosia. When comparing to the former PET studies, there was an inverse correlation between areas of hypometabolism observed in the FDG-PET and increased uptake in the GTP-PET study, irrespective of beta-amyloid distribution (Fig. 3).

## Diagnosis

Multidomain mild cognitive impairment due to early onset Alzheimer's disease (AD).

## Discussion

The case presented here shows that the etiological diagnostic process in some patients with an atypical presentation of cognitive impairment can be challenging and may be difficult to achieve

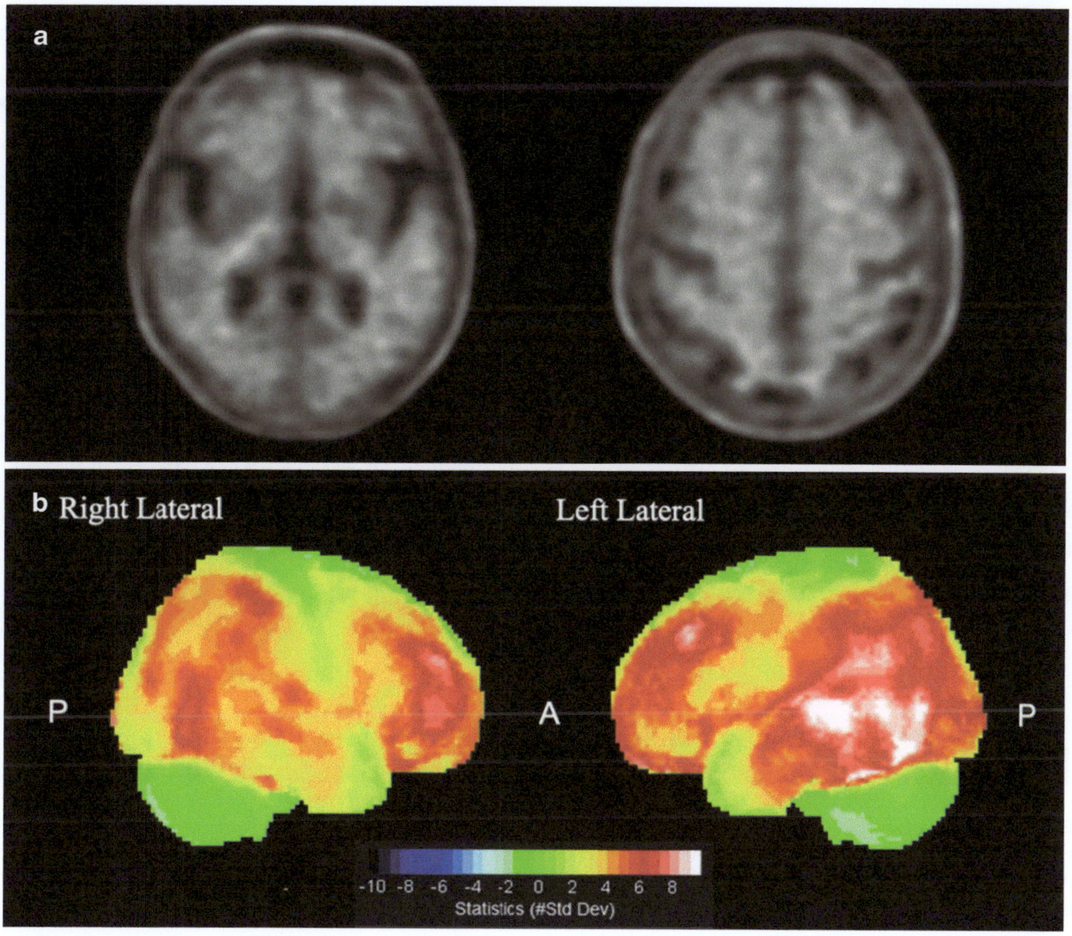


**Fig. 2** PET/CT with [$^{18}$F]Florbetaben (amyloid). (**a**) Sequential axial slices indicating an increase of cortical β-amyloid load. (**b**) Comparison with the normal database in surface projections (3D-SSP; Syngo.via database comparison, Siemens). Cortical areas with a significant increase of β-amyloid burden are shown in red (>2 SD)

based exclusively on the standard evaluation. Specifically, patients under 65 years of age have a greater cognitive reserve that might limit the assessment of the diagnosis. Additionally, the presence of a psychiatric comorbidity (depressive disorder) that could interfere with the cognitive decline. Furthermore, the clinical phenotype is also atypical, highlighting the progression of the visuospatial and visuoperceptual impairment in the context of a multidomain MCI.

However, a precise etiological diagnosis is necessary to define the prognosis and make a therapeutic decision or, when appropriate, to select patients to be included in clinical trials that may offer a therapeutic alternative in the absence of a curative treatment for AD.

The new criteria for the diagnosis of MCI due to AD according to the National Institute of Aging Alzheimer Association (NIA-AA), and the criteria for AD (IWG-2 criteria for AD), recognize the importance of biomarkers to facilitate the etiological diagnosis [2, 3]. The imaging biomarkers are very useful for the early and differential diagnosis of neurodegenerative diseases associated with dementia. Among the most widely used biomarkers in neuroimaging are amyloid PET, which identifies neuritic plaques deposition into the brain, and FDG-PET, which assesses neuronal glucose

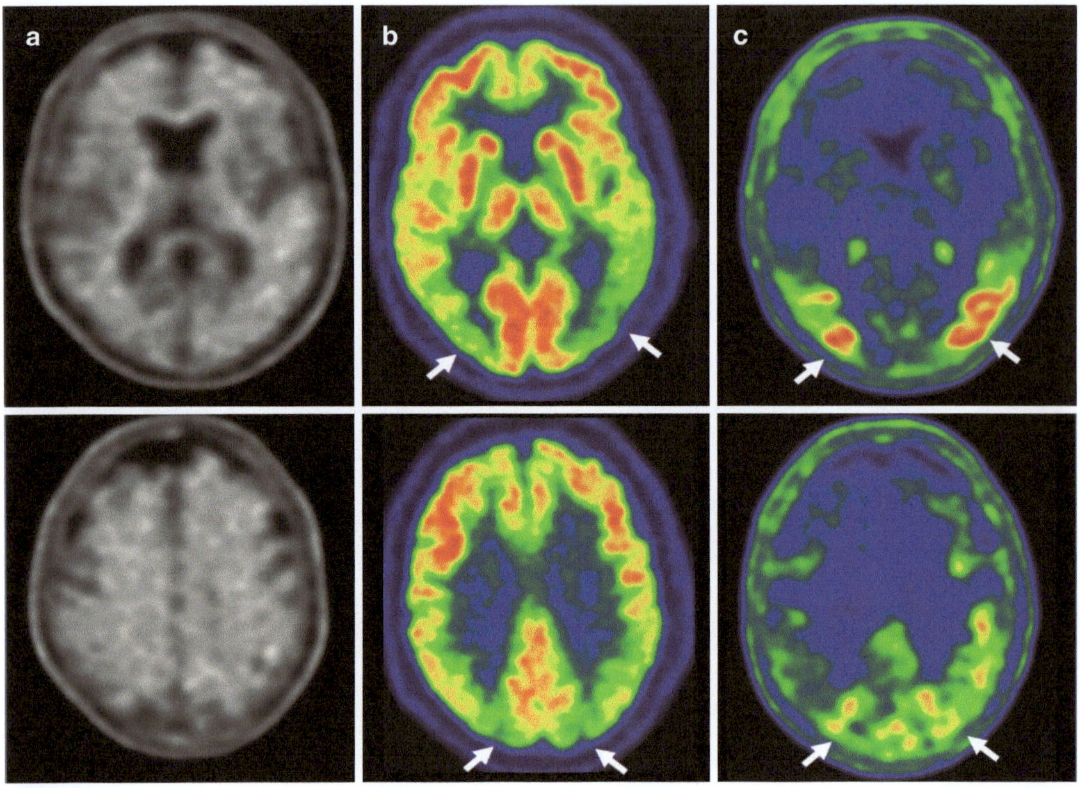


**Fig. 3** Brain PET Biomarkers. (**a**) PET/CT [$^{18}$F] Florbetaben (amyloid), increase of cortical β-amyloid neuritic plaques that do not correlate with the other biomarkers. (**b**) [$^{18}$F]FDG hypometabolism of the predominantly left parieto-temporal region and the lateral region of the bilateral occipital cortex. (**c**) [$^{18}$F]GTP1 uptake showing tau pathology in the areas where hypometabolism of FDG is observed (arrows)

metabolism, providing complementary information on neurodegeneration.

Amyloid PET allows a noninvasive visualization of AD pathology in the brain with a sensitivity of 91–98% and specificity of 87–100% in patients with AD confirmed by autopsy [4–6]. This imaging technique has not contraindications or side effects beyond exceptional injection site irritation and flushing. Additionally, the variability of the amyloid PET interpretation across centers and individuals is low [4, 7]. On the other hand, FDG-PET allows the visualization of the location and extent of neuronal dysfunction, which helps for making a differential diagnosis between neurodegenerative diseases or their clinical variants, and for predicting short-term outcomes in MCI subjects or staging neurodegenerative processes [7].

Tau-PET shows the density and distribution of tau neurofibrillary tangles in patients with cognitive impairment due to AD [8]. The radiotracer distribution observed in the tau-PET scan in this case was unrelated to the amyloid plaques location, but matched the areas of hypometabolism shown by the FDG-PET. Interestingly, the hypometabolism and tau burden involved the visual association area (temporo-occipital and parieto-occipital regions) and correlated with the visual agnosia in the presence of a significant increase of amyloid in the brain. This clinical and imaging pattern is highly suggestive of a posterior cortical atrophy variant of AD.

Nevertheless, tau-PET offers some advantages over FDG-PET as tau pathology appeared prior to the neurodegenerative changes, it has an excellent correlation with the clinical phenotype, and blood glucose levels, functional diaschisis or comorbidities do not influence it. Recently, the US Food and Drug Administration approved the clinical use of a PET-tau biomarker (Flortaucipir, Tauvid®). This fact constitutes a great step forward in the development of biomarkers that help clinicians give an accurate diagnosis in early stages of complex cases of neurodegenerative disorders, facilitating decision-making and patient selection for clinical trials of new therapeutic lines.

## Conclusions

Current neuroimaging biomarkers facilitate an early and accurate characterization of the etiological diagnosis in atypical clinical presentations and in the presence of comorbidities, Furthermore, molecular imaging biomarkers are essential for selecting patients who may benefit from specific investigational treatments. The development of tau-PET imaging offers advantages over standard neurodegeneration biomarkers for the differential diagnosis between neurodegenerative conditions associated with dementia.

## References

1. Barthel H, Gertz HJ, Dresel S, Peters O, Bartenstein P, Buerger K, et al. Cerebral amyloid-β PET with florbetaben (18F) in patients with Alzheimer's disease and healthy controls: a multicentre phase 2 diagnostic study. Lancet Neurol. 2011;10(5):424–35.
2. Dubois B, Feldman HH, Jacova C, Hampel H, Molinuevo JL, Blennow K, et al. Advancing research diagnostic criteria for Alzheimer's disease: the IWG-2 criteria. Lancet Neurol. 2014;13:614–29.
3. Albert MS, DeKosky ST, Dickson D, Dubois B, Feldman HH, Fox NC, et al. The diagnosis of mild cognitive impairment due to Alzheimer's disease: recommendations from the National Institute on Aging-Alzheimer's Association workgroups on diagnostic guidelines for Alzheimer's disease. Alzheimers Dement. 2011;7:270–9.
4. Clark CM, Pontecorvo MJ, Beach TG, Bedell BJ, Coleman RE, Doraiswamy PM, et al. Cerebral PET with florbetapir compared with neuropathology at autopsy for detection of neuritic amyloid-β plaques: a prospective cohort study. Lancet Neurol. 2012;11:669–78.
5. Sabri O, Sabbagh MN, Seibyl J, et al. Florbetaben PET imaging to detect amyloid beta plaques in Alzheimer's disease: phase 3 study. Alzheimers Dement. 2015;11:964–74.
6. Salloway S, Gamez JE, Singh U, et al. Performance of [18F]flutemetamol amyloid imaging against the neuritic plaque component of CERAD and the current (2012) NIA-AA recommendations for the neuropathologic diagnosis of Alzheimer's disease. Alzheimers Dement. 2017;9:25–34.
7. Chételat G, Arbizu J, Barthel H, Garibotto V, Law I, Morbelli S, et al. Amyloid-PET and 18F-FDG-PET in the diagnostic investigation of Alzheimer's disease and other dementias. Lancet Neurol. 2020;19(11):951–62. https://linkinghub.elsevier.com/retrieve/pii/S1474442220303148.
8. First BH, Tau PET. Tracer approved: toward accurate in vivo diagnosis of Alzheimer disease. J Nucl Med. 2020;61:1409–10.

# Case 3: Alzheimer's Disease—Behavioral Variant

Silvia Morbelli, Matteo Pardini, and Flavio Nobili

## Introduction

The term 'frontal variant' of Alzheimer's disease (fvAD) refers to a rare phenotype underpinned by amyloid plaque and neurofibrillary tangle pathology but in which behavioral and/or dysexecutive deficits predominate.

The clinical presentation of fvAD may mimic that of behavioral variant frontotemporal dementia (bvFTD). Therefore about 80% of patients with fvAD meet the clinical criteria for possible bvFTD and, conversely, 10–40% of patients with a clinical diagnosis of bvFTD actually disclose AD pathology by means of either in vivo (CSF, amyloid PET) or *postmortem* assessments.

Typically, in such behavioral/dysexecutive presentation of AD the severity of behavioral symptoms is lower than in bvFTD, but patients are more cognitively impaired, often showing similar memory deficit as in typical AD and worse executive functioning than patients with either bvFTD or typical AD. The prominent frontal syndrome in fvAD is likely the result of a selective neurodegeneration in frontal control networks, but neurodegeneration usually spares frontal lobe and mostly involves the temporoparietal regions. Therefore, structural MRI provides useful information to distinguish fvAD from frontotemporal lobar degeneration (FTLD) whose atrophy pattern typically affects anterior brain regions.

When structural MRI is not fully able to elucidate the regional pattern of neurodegeneration in the earliest stages, PET with fluorine-18 fluorodeoxyglucose ([$^{18}$F]FDG PET) can detect neuronal injury and the distribution of hypometabolism, which though closely overlaps between fvAD and FTLD by affecting medial and orbital frontal areas. Therefore, if available, amyloid-specific biomarkers (PET or CSF) are proposed to confirm or rule out AD pathology as the causative etiology in those patients with a behavioral or a dysexecutive clinical presentation. Although, concerns persist that patients with FTLD pathology may rarely have false positivity for amyloid PET due to the coexistence of Pick bodies or TDP-43 aggregates and Alzheimer's pathology.

S. Morbelli (✉)
IRCCS Ospedale Policlinico San Martino, Genoa, Italy

Nuclear Medicine Unit, Department of Health Sciences, University of Genoa, Genoa, Italy
e-mail: silviadaniela.morbelli@hsanmartino.it

M. Pardini · F. Nobili
IRCCS Ospedale Policlinico San Martino, Genoa, Italy

Department of Neuroscience, Rehabilitation, Ophthalmology, Genetics, Maternal and Child Health (DINOGMI), University of Genoa, Genoa, Italy



A. Varrone et al. (eds.), *Clinical Nuclear Medicine in Neurology*,
https://doi.org/10.1007/978-3-030-83598-9_3

## Case Presentation

- A 68-year-old Caucasian woman with no previous history of psychiatric disease.
- The patient developed anxiety, irritability as well as mild memory and dysexecutive complaints, with some impairment in the instrumental activities of daily living (IADL).
- No familiarity for neurological diseases and, apart from the removal of a thyroid nodule 15 years before, she only had undergone surgery for titanium hip replacement which was complicated by delirium during the hospitalization in the recent months.
- Neurological exam and standard blood tests were unremarkable.
- The standard neuropsychological assessment revealed a significant impairment in memory (Corsi and Digit Span, Rey Auditory Verbal Learning tests), executive functions and attention (Trail making test, digit symbol, stroop color and stroop color word), visual abilities (clock drawing test) and semantic fluency, with a score of 26/30 at the synoptic Mini-Mental State examination (MMSE).
- Electroencephalography (EEG) registered a slowing down of mean frequencies and brain magnetic resonance imaging (MRI) disclosed atrophy of medial temporal and posterior parietal areas, as well as of polar temporal and frontal cortices (Fig. 1).
- The multidomain mild cognitive impairment (mdMCI), with both amnestic and dysexecutive presentation, and the atrophic pattern involving medial temporal and posterior parietal areas found at the morphological evaluation (MRI) initially led the clinician to the suspicion of Alzheimer's disease (MCI-AD).
- [$^{18}$F]FDG PET was performed to confirm the clinical suspicion and showed hypometabolism in bilateral polar and ventral-lateral frontal cortices, as well as in left insula, anterior and middle cingulate and with a lesser extent even in posterior parietal areas, which was consistent either with fvAD or FTLD pattern (see Fig. 2).
- To firmly distinguish between the two conditions—i.e., AD and FTLD—the patient was submitted to PET with amyloid-specific tracer ([$^{18}$F]Florbetapir) disclosing a diffuse amyloidotic process in the brain (Fig. 3).
- The clinical presentation, the involvement of posterior areas unveiled by both morphological and functional imaging and the final evidence of diffuse brain amyloidosis suggested the diagnosis of MCI due to a frontal variant of AD (fvAD).
- She was treated with a cholinesterase inhibitor (donepezil) as well as with atypical neuroleptics and antidepressant to manage the behavioral and psychological symptoms which had worsened during the follow-up.
- She converted to dementia after 4 years. At the last available visit (8 years from diagnosis) she had a severe cognitive deficit with speech impairment (MMSE unperformable, Clinical Dementia rating scale 4) and behavioral symptoms which only partially benefit from antipsychotic drugs.

## Imaging Findings

- Brain MRI (Fig. 1)
- [$^{18}$F]FDG PET (Fig. 2)
- Amyloid PET (Fig. 3)

**Take Home Messages**

- fvAD is a quite rare variant of AD which is often difficultly distinguished from other conditions with behavioral and dysexecutive presentation such as bvFTD.
- A combination of early cognitive deficits, including poor memory and executive performance, and an intermediate behavioral profile can help to differentiate fvAD and bvFTD at a clinical level.

- Brain atrophy predominantly affects temporoparietal cortex in both classical AD and fvAD compared to bvFTD in which anterior areas are mostly involved.
- The pattern of hypometabolism is often similar in fvAD and FTLD, but semi-quantitative tools for the analysis of PET images may be helpful. The involvement of precuneus/posterior cingulate in addition to frontotemporal lobes may be a useful tool to suggest Alzheimer's pathology (fvAD) rather than FTLD, in which posterior areas are usually spared in the earliest stages.
- The use of a pathologic biomarker of amyloidosis (amyloid PET or CSF Aβ-amyloid) is proposed to further sustain the diagnosis of fvAD, even if some cautious is needed due to the risk of false positivity of the amyloid PET scan in FTD patients.
- Long-term prognosis is worse and need of assistance is higher in patients with fvAD than FTLD but acetylcholinesterase inhibitors may be helpful.

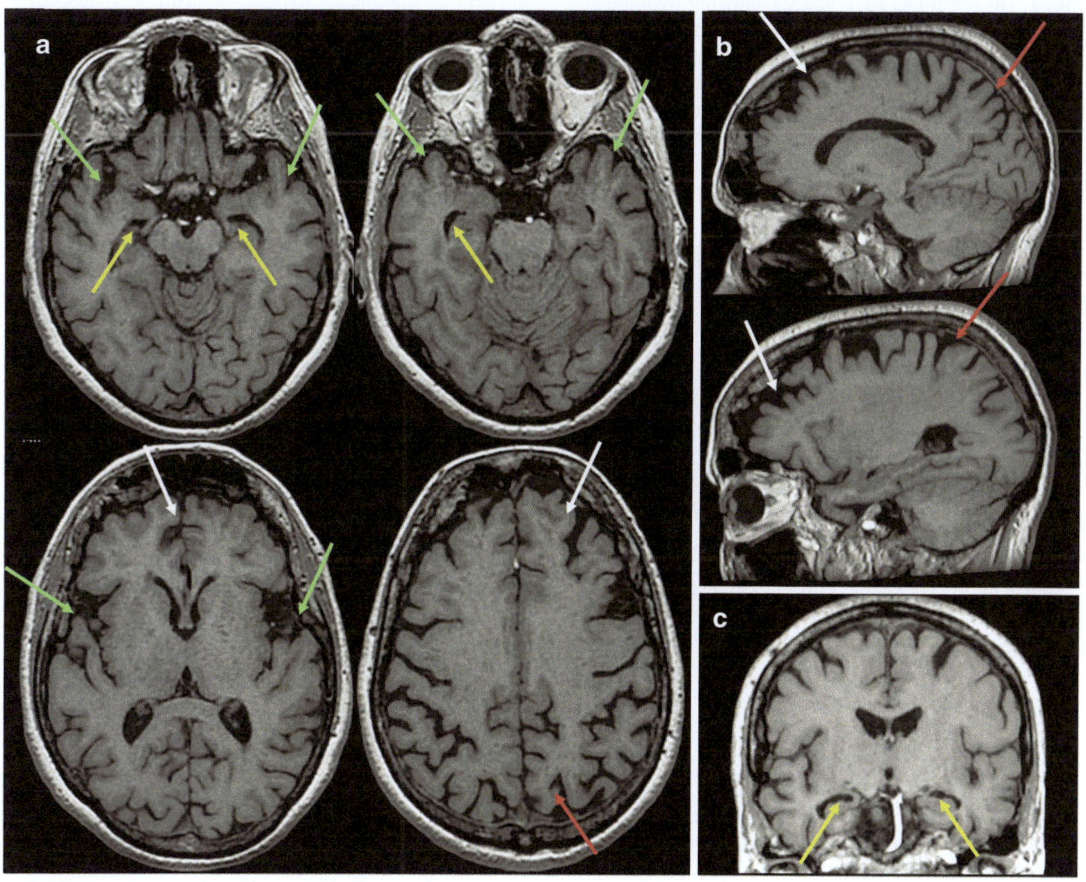


**Fig. 1** Axial (**a**), sagittal (**b**) and coronal (**c**) T1-weighted MRI images showing atrophy in mesial temporal lobe (yellow arrows) and parietal and posterior cingulate areas (red arrows) with enlargement of occipital horns of the lateral ventricles, but also in frontal (white arrows) and polar and lateral temporal lobes (right > left) (green arrows)

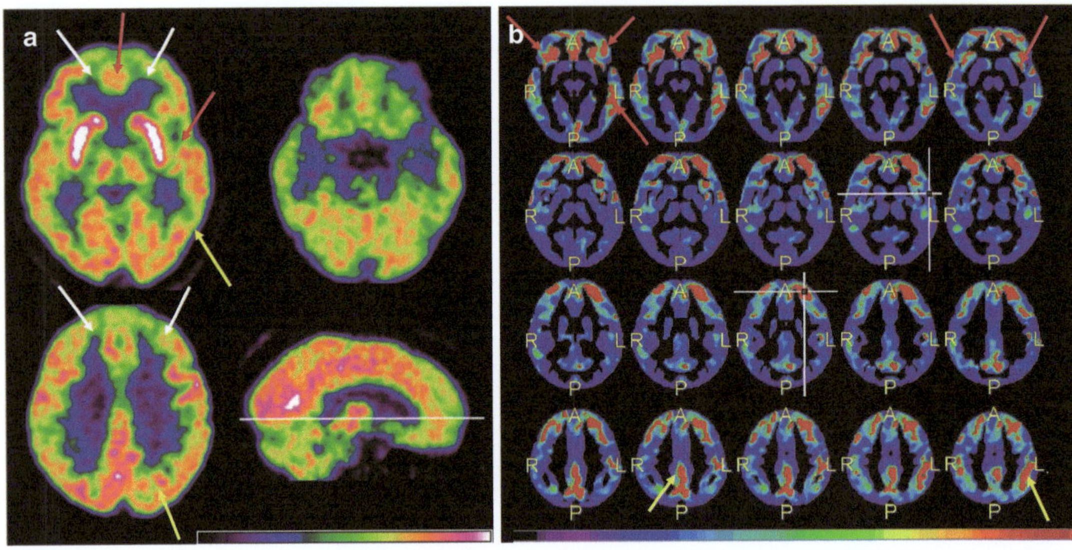


**Fig. 2** (**a**) [$^{18}$F]FDG PET images showing hypometabolism in bilateral polar and ventral-lateral frontal cortices (white arrows), as well as in left insula, anterior and middle cingulate (red arrows) and asymmetric metabolism (left<right) in posterior parietal areas (yellow arrows). (**b**) Results of whole brain voxel-wise analysis with respect to age-matched controls following the method described by Herholz et al. 2002 (cfr suggested readings). In red color clusters of significant hypometabolism with respect to controls are displayed in both polar and ventral-lateral frontal areas, as well as in insular, anterior and middle cingulate, polar and lateral temporal areas (red arrows). Voxel-wise analysis also evidenced a significant hypometabolism in posterior parietal cortex and in precuneus/posterior cingulate with respect to controls (yellow arrows), which was less evident in visual analysis

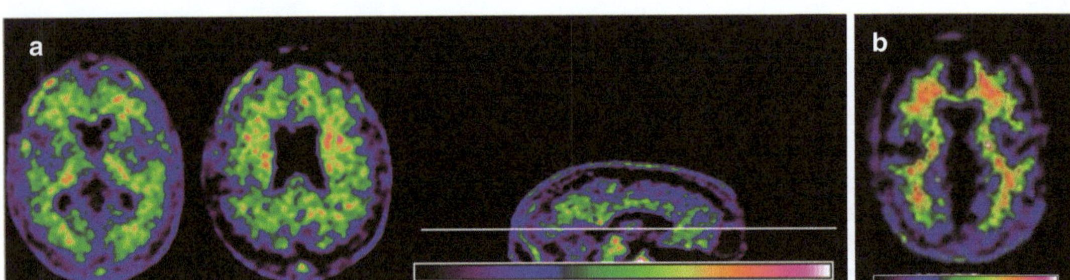


**Fig. 3** (**a**) The amyloid PET displays an increased [$^{18}$F] Florbetapir uptake in the cortical cerebral grey matter, with higher intensity in the frontal and parietal lobes. The scan is positive and is consistent with the presence of moderate to frequent neuritic beta-amyloid plaques in the brain. (**b**) An example of a negative amyloid PET scan in which the [$^{18}$F]Florbetapir uptake is restricted to the lipophilic white matter without involving cortical areas

## Suggested Readings


Beach TG, Monsell SE, Phillips LE, Kukull W. Accuracy of the clinical diagnosis of Alzheimer disease at National Institute on Aging Alzheimer Disease Centers, 2005–2010. J Neuropathol Exp Neurol. 2012;71:266–73.

Herholz K, Salmon E, Perani D, et al. Discrimination between Alzheimer dementia and controls by automated analysis of multicenter FDG PET. NeuroImage. 2002;17:302–16.

Hof PR, Bouras C, Perl DP, Morrison JH. Quantitative neuropathologic analysis of Pick's disease cases: cortical distribution of Pick bodies and coexistence with Alzheimer's disease. Acta Neuropathol. 1994;87:115–24.

Rabinovici GD, Rosen HJ, Alkalay A, et al. Amyloid vs FDG-PET in the differential diagnosis of AD and FTLD. Neurology. 2011;77(23):2034–42.

Wolk DA. Amyloid imaging in atypical presentations of Alzheimer's disease. Curr Neurol Neurosci Rep. 2013;13:412.

Womack KB, Diaz-Arrastia R, Aizenstein HJ, et al. Temporoparietal hypometabolism in frontotemporal lobar degeneration and associated imaging diagnostic errors. Arch Neurol. 2011;68:329–37.

# Case 4: Parkinson's Disease with Onset as Mild Cognitive Impairment (MCI)

Federico Massa and Silvia Morbelli

## Introduction

Mild cognitive impairment (MCI) can be detected at any time in subjects with Parkinson's disease (PD) even in the earliest stages of the disease. MCI has also been described as a possible—albeit uncommon—presenting symptom of PD ~~(Mas~~ and indeed the construct of PD with cognitive presentation is contained in the current diagnostic criteria.

The clinical approach to the cognitive presentations of PD is challenging and biomarkers are needed to identify both those MCI which are underpinned by an alpha-synucleinopathy and those subjects with a high-risk of developing cognitive deterioration in the short-to-midterm. As for the neuropsychological profile, patient mainly shows a non-amnestic profile, but also memory can be affected as part of a multidomain MCI. Structural neuroimaging may guide clinicians in the differential diagnosis when either vascular damage or regional atrophy is evident, thus suggesting conditions such as vascular cognitive impairment, Alzheimer's disease (AD) or frontotemporal lobe degeneration (FTLD). However, it can also be the case that PD-MCI patients actually disclose mild medial temporal lobe (MTL) atrophy as well as a significant memory impairment. In such situation the distinction between PD-MCI and MCI-AD is rather subtle, thus leading to a misdiagnosis. A deep investigation of motor and non-motor symptoms, which might be overlooked or absent at the earliest stages, and the use of diagnostic tools such as electroencephalography and functional imaging can finally disclose those typical features which allow to suggest that MCI is due to PD or, more generally to a Lewy-body disease (LBD). Indeed, the construct of PD-MCI overlaps that of dementia with Lewy bodies (DLB) in its prodromal (or MCI) stage. As several motor and non-motor symptoms are shared, the two conditions are considered as two extremities of the same LBD spectrum. Biomarker investigation and clinical follow-up are needed to subsequently clarify the evolutive trajectory within the LBD spectrum.

## Case Presentation

– A 70-year-old Caucasian man with previous history of resection of prostate cancer and mild hypertension and dyslipidemia. No

F. Massa
Department of Neuroscience, Rehabilitation, Ophthalmology, Genetics, Maternal and Child Health (DINOGMI), University of Genoa, Genoa, Italy

S. Morbelli (✉)
IRCCS Ospedale Policlinico San Martino, Genoa, Italy

Nuclear Medicine Unit, Department of Health Sciences, University of Genoa, Genoa, Italy
e-mail: silviadaniela.morbelli@hsanmartino.it


A. Varrone et al. (eds.), *Clinical Nuclear Medicine in Neurology*,
https://doi.org/10.1007/978-3-030-83598-9_4

familiarity for neurological or psychiatric conditions.

- The patient referred to a neurologist due to memory and attention difficulties, loss of interests and sociality, without any functional impairment.
- Neurological exam and standard blood tests were unremarkable.
- The standard neuropsychological assessment revealed a significant impairment in several domains, i.e., executive functions and attention (Trail making test, stroop color and stroop color word), memory (Rey Auditory Verbal Learning and Babcock story recall test) and language (phonemic verbal fluency in particular), with a score of 27/30 at the synoptic Mini-Mental State examination (MMSE).
- Electroencephalography (EEG) registered a slowing down of mean frequencies (7–8 Hz) and brain magnetic resonance imaging (MRI) disclosed few vascular lesions in subcortical white matter and mild cortical loss in temporal, frontal, and posterior parietal areas (left>right) (Fig. 1).
- As the clinical presentation was atypical (both amnestic and dysexecutive presentation) and the morphological imaging poorly informative, the patient was submitted to [$^{18}$F]FDG PET which showed a moderate metabolic asymmetry in temporoparietal areas (left<right) (Fig. 2a).
- The multidomain mild cognitive impairment (mdMCI) and the posterior pattern of atrophy and hypometabolism suggested a tentative diagnosis of MCI due to Alzheimer's disease (MCI-AD), therefore treatment with cholinesterase inhibitor (rivastigmine) was started.
- The patient remained cognitively steady during the 3-year follow-up (MMSE 28/30), then slowness of movements, hypomimia and hypophonia occurred, along with mild depression and sleep behavior disorder (acting the dream, falls from bed), which though had been occurred for many years but never reported or deeply investigated. Also, constipation had become more severe.
- At neurological examination right-predominant akinetic-rigid syndrome and hyposmia were then detected, but no tremor of orthostatic hypotension. REM behavior disorder (RBD) was also registered by means of polysomnography, thus suggesting a Lewy-body disease.
- This clinical hypothesis was confirmed by the significant nigrostriatal impairment in bilateral putamen (left>right), detected by means of [$^{123}$I]FP-CIT-SPECT (Fig. 3). The LBD diagnosis was further sustained by the RT-Quic analysis performed in nasal brushing which specifically detected alpha-synuclein protein.
- Response to treatment with iMAO inhibitor (rasagiline), dopamine-agonist (ropinirole), and levodopa/carbidopa was significant. Rivastigmine was also maintained to treat the cognitive disorder.
- After 5 years from baseline an FDG PET scan was performed and disclosed a significant worsening of brain metabolism in bilateral posterior parietal, lateral temporal and occipital regions, and also hypometabolic changes in precuneus/posterior cingulate cortex (Fig. 2b).
- At the last available follow-up visit (10 years from the baseline) he had mild dementia (MMSE 18/30), rare visual hallucinations and needed assistance for activities of daily living. He also needed support for walking due to the risk of falls because of the worsening of akinetic-rigid syndrome and unbalance.
- Levodopa response, slow progression to dementia and the substantial lack of behavior and psychological symptoms until the latest stages of the disease further supported the diagnosis of PD-MCI, lately converted to PD-dementia, rather than of DLB.

## Imaging Findings

- Brain MRI (Fig. 1)
- [$^{18}$F]FDG PET, visual analysis (Fig. 2)
- [$^{123}$I]FP-CIT-SPECT (Fig. 3)
- [$^{18}$F]FDG PET, semiquantitative analysis (Fig. 4)

**Teaching Points**

- Parkinson's disease (PD) is one of the possible etiologies of MCI, and MCI in PD may even precede the onset of motor impairment in a non-negligible part of patients.
- MCI is hardly attributed to PD when a clear motor syndrome is absent and if it differs from the expected non-amnestic profile.
- Brain MRI can support the differential diagnosis between MCI due to AD or PD, but a certain degree of atrophy in medial temporal or posterior parietal lobes is sometimes shared by the two conditions.
- The pattern of hypometabolism affecting posterior areas in [$^{18}$F]FDG PET can be misleading in the differential diagnosis between AD and LBD in their earliest stages. However, the typical pattern of metabolism affecting parietooccipital lobes is a consistent finding during the course of LBD and matches with the severity of cognitive impairment from MCI to dementia stages.
- When motor symptoms are undetectable, a deep investigation of the typical non-motor symptoms, i.e., RBD, constipation and hyposmia, is helpful to suggest an MCI due to a Lewy-body disease (LBD).
- The cholinergic deficit is higher in LBD than in AD and parallels both the slowing down of mean frequencies at EEG and the cognitive impairment which thus benefits from cholinesterase inhibitors.
- Biomarker investigation and clinical follow-up allow to clarify the evolutive trajectory within the LBD spectrum and the risk of evolution to dementia in the short-to-midterm.

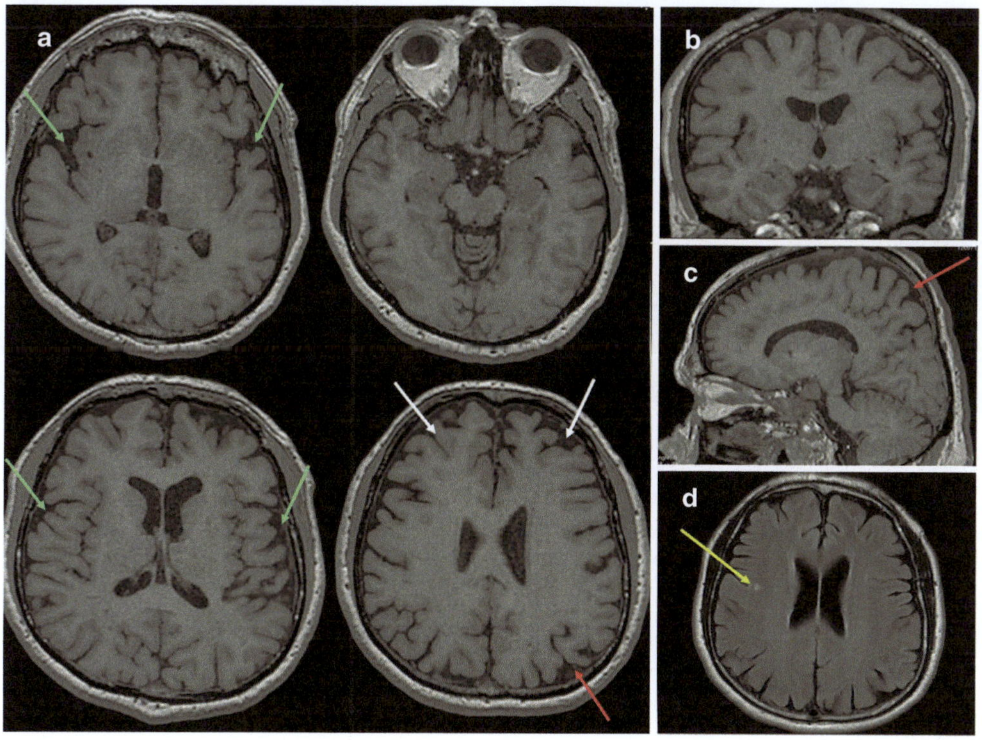


**Fig. 1** Axial (**a**), sagittal (**b**) and coronal (**c**) T1-weighted MRI images showing mild atrophy in temporal (green arrows), frontal (white arrows) and posterior parietal areas (red arrows) (left > right) (green arrows). (**d**) Example of vascular lesion in subcortical white matter displayed by axial T2 Flair sequence (yellow arrow)

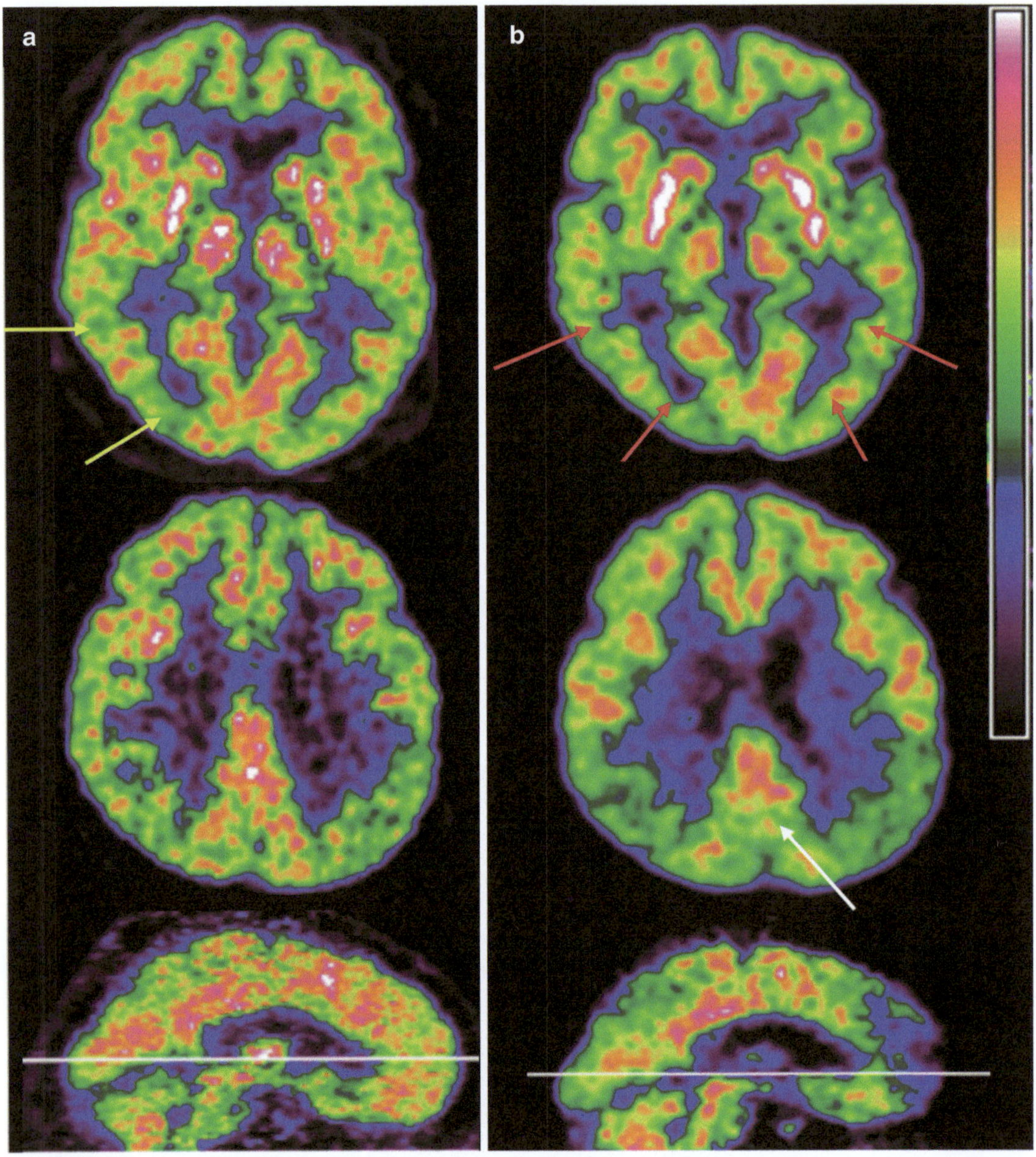


**Fig. 2** (**a**) [$^{18}$F]FDG PET images at baseline showing asymmetric metabolism (left < right) in lateral temporal and posterior parietal regions (yellow arrows). (**b**) Images of the FDG PET scan performed after 5 years from baseline disclosing a significant worsening of brain metabolism affecting bilateral posterior parietal, lateral temporal and occipital regions (red arrows). A less severe hypometabolism (left < right) is also displayed in precuneus/posterior cingulate cortex (white arrow)

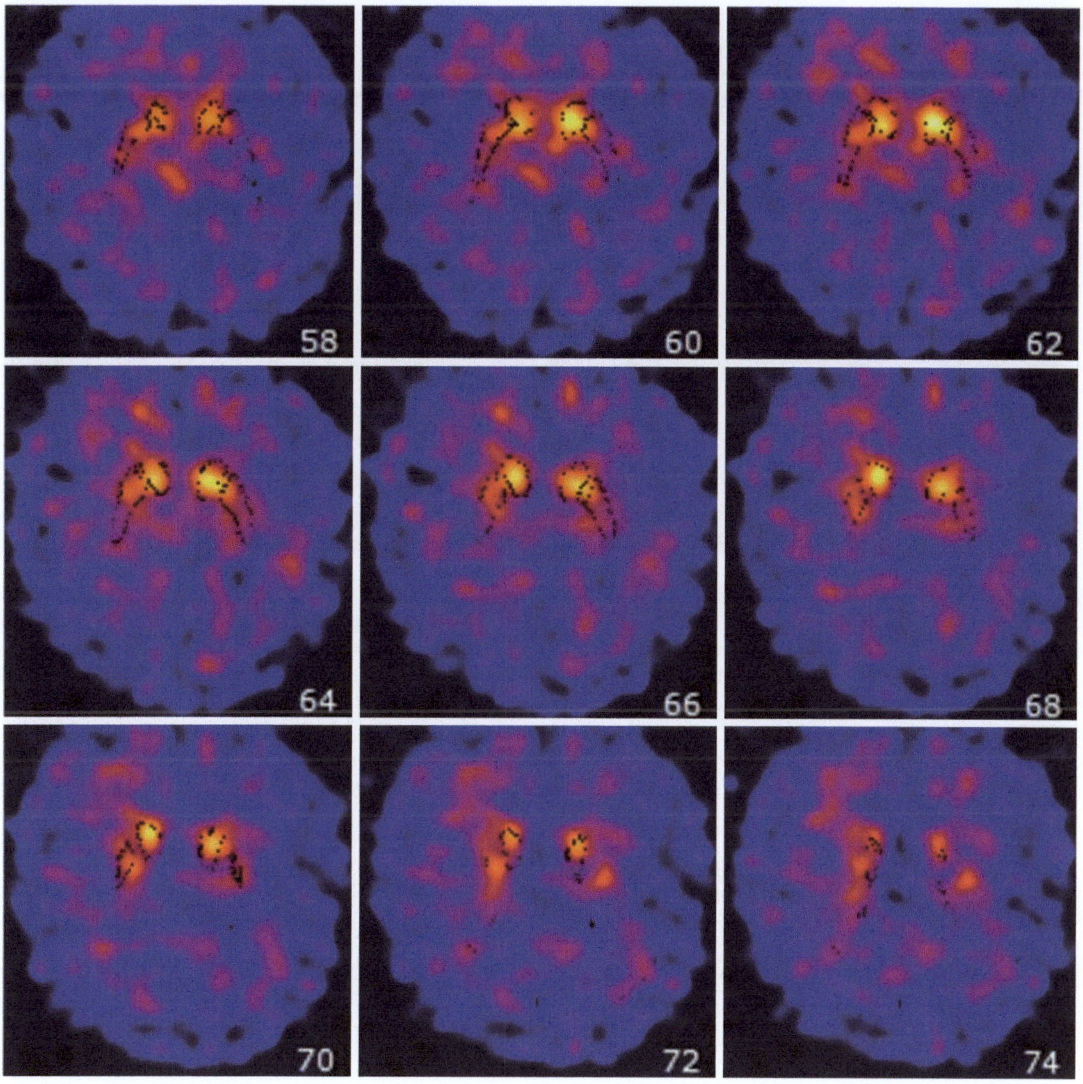


**Fig. 3** SPECT images showing a severe dopaminergic nigrostriatal denervation in bilateral putamen (left > right)

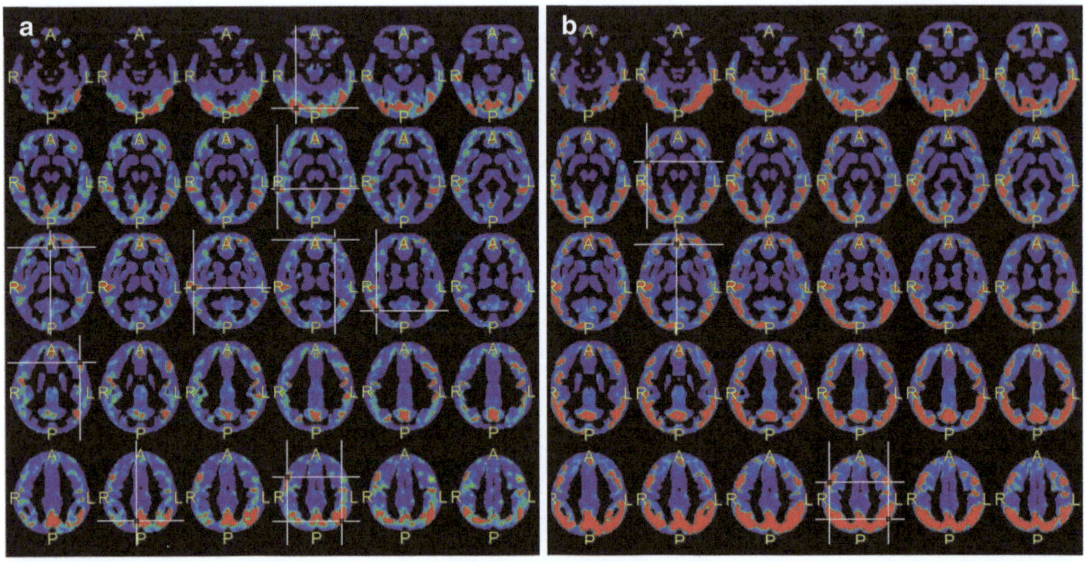


**Fig. 4** Results of whole brain voxel-wise analysis with respect to age-matched controls following the method described by Herholz et al. (2002) (cfr suggested readings). In red color clusters of significant hypometabolism with respect to controls are displayed. A significant spreading of hypometabolism is evident in the [[18]F]FDG PET scan performed after 5 years from initial presentation (**b**) than that at baseline (**a**), especially in parietal-occipital regions and, even if with as lesser extent, also in lateral temporal and frontal areas

## Suggested Reading


Berg D, Postuma RB, Bloem B. Time to redefine PD? Introductory statement of the MDS Task Force on the definition of Parkinson's disease. Mov Disord. 2014;29:454–62.

Bohnen NI, Albin RL. The cholinergic system and Parkinson disease. Behav Brain Res. 2011;221: 564–73.

Fairfoul G, McGuire LI, Pal S, et al. Alpha-synuclein RT-QuIC in the CSF of patients with alpha-synucleinopathies. Ann Clin Transl Neurol. 2016;3:812–8.

Massa F, Meli R, Grazzini M, et al. Utility of quantitative EEG in early Lewy body disease. Parkinsonism Relat Disord. 2020;75:70–5.

Reingold JL, Morgan JC, Sethi KD. Rivastigmine for the treatment of dementia associated with Parkinson's disease. Neuropsychiatr Dis Treat. 2007;6:775–83.

# Case 5: Parkinson's Disease with Vascular Abnormalities

Elsmarieke van de Giessen

## Clinical Background

A 63-year-old man was referred to a tertiary center for diagnostics of tremor, balance and walking problems, and tendency to dystonia. Since 1.5 years he was complaining about shaking movements, including chattering jaws, trembling legs and a tremor of his hands (left more than right). The hand tremor usually occurred when reaching out for something, but not at rest. This interfered with eating soup for example or sending text messages. Furthermore, patient reported that his balance was disturbed. He regularly had to keep himself from falling, but remembered falling only once. He also felt that he had more difficulty walking with sometimes episodes where he could not walk straight. Since 2 months, the patient also noticed that he was slower. In addition, he mentioned that his smell was nearly gone.

Patient reported no cognitive problems or mood disturbances, although he started living more in his own world according to his son. He had no clinically relevant medical history, did not use any medication, and did not drink alcohol. There was no family history of neurologic disorders.

A movement disorder specialist found the following symptoms at neurologic examination. Patient had a stiff walking pattern with reduced arm swing on the right side. The pull-test was abnormal indicating postural instability. There was subtle global bradykinesia (right more than left) and some rigidity of the arms (right more than left). There was no rest tremor, but a mild postural tremor (left more than right), that worsened at intention. When the left index finger was brought toward the thumb, there was a coarse tremor of the left hand, which disappeared when the patient was distracted. No tremor of the jaws. Patient had mild mirror dystonia of the left hand. Reflexes, coordination, and sensibility were normal.

Plasma laboratory findings (including among others thyroid function, vitamin B12, magnesium, M-protein, and ferritin) were conducted in the referring hospital and were normal.

An MRI scan of the brain of the patient was acquired in the referring hospital in the previous three months. There were large confluent white matter hyperintensities periventricular and in the deep white matter in both hemispheres (Fazekas score 3), which are of presumed vascular origin. In addition, there were multiple lacunar infarctions, amongst others in the caudate nucleus and putamen on the right and in the semioval center. There were no cortical infarctions and no microbleeds. Furthermore, there was no abnormal atrophy pattern, there were no signs of atypical parkinsonisms and there were no clinically relevant other findings.

E. van de Giessen (✉)
Department of Radiology and Nuclear Medicine, Amsterdam UMC, location VUmc, Amsterdam, The Netherlands



A. Varrone et al. (eds.), *Clinical Nuclear Medicine in Neurology*,
https://doi.org/10.1007/978-3-030-83598-9_5

In summary, the neurologist identified a task-specific tremor of the left hand, which was suspected for a functional tremor. Secondly, there was hyposmia and possible rigidity and reduced arm swing of the right arm without bradykinesia, which may indicate but are insufficient for a probable diagnosis of Parkinson's Disease (PD). Furthermore, the MRI scan showed a large vascular-ischemic burden, which may contribute to the symptoms. To further clarify the underlying etiology, the neurologist requested a dopamine transporter single photon emission computed tomography (SPECT) scan.

## Dopamine Transporter SPECT Scan

A dopamine transporter SPECT scan of the brain was acquired in the patient according to a standard protocol that has been described in detail previously [1]. In short, the patient was injected with 116 MBq [$^{123}$I]FP-CIT (GE Healthcare) and scanned 3 hours post-injection on an InSPira system, which is a brain-dedicated SPECT system that differs from conventional SPECT scanners with respect to hardware configuration and scanning geometry resulting in increased spatial resolution. The detector ring consists of two clamshells, each containing 12 (focusing) fan-beam collimators. The head of the patient was positioned along the orbitomeatal line. A proprietary iterative reconstruction algorithm (with 60 iterations) was used to reconstruct the data into 3D images. This iterative reconstruction algorithm is based on a maximum a posteriori (MAP) estimation and includes a point spread function (PSF). An adult head CT template was manually aligned and used for attenuation correction.

Both visual and semi-quantitative analysis was performed by an experienced reader. Semi-quantitative analysis was performed automatically using BRASS (BRASS™, HERMES Medical, Sweden), as described previously [1]. BRASS registers the patient data to a template with volumes of interest for right and left caudate nucleus, putamen, whole striatum and occipital cortex. The ratio of counts in the region of interest (caudate nucleus, putamen, whole putamen) subtracted with the counts in the reference region (occipital cortex) divided by the counts in the reference region (occipital cortex). The semiquantitative results were compared to a locally acquired database of age-matched healthy controls resulting in calculation of *Z*-scores.

The images showed reduced binding in the putamen bilaterally, left more than right. There was visually normal binding in the left caudate nucleus. On the right side, there was reduced binding in the posterior putamen and lower irregular binding in the caudate nucleus and anterior putamen. When correlating these images with the MRI scan, the irregular binding could be explained by the lacunar infarction at this location.

The binding ratios as determined with semi-quantitative analysis were: right caudate 1.55, left caudate 2.04, right putamen 1.21, and left putamen 1.35. The *Z*-scores confirmed reduced binding in the putamen on both sides (left −2.7; right −2.8). The *Z*-score for the right caudate nucleus was also very low (−2.1). For the left caudate nucleus the *Z*-score was low (−1.8), but considered within normal limits (> −2.0). The putamen/caudate ratios are 0.78 for the right side and 0.66 for the left side. These results are strongly suggestive of nigrostriatal neurodegeneration in combination with reduced binding due to a vascular lesion in the striatum on the right side.

## Conclusion

The patient presented with an asymmetric hypokinetic rigid syndrome which, based on the symptoms, the DAT SPECT and MRI scan, was diagnosed as probable idiopathic PD with comorbid cerebrovascular disease (Figs. 1 and 2). The tremor of the left hand was interpreted as a functional tremor.

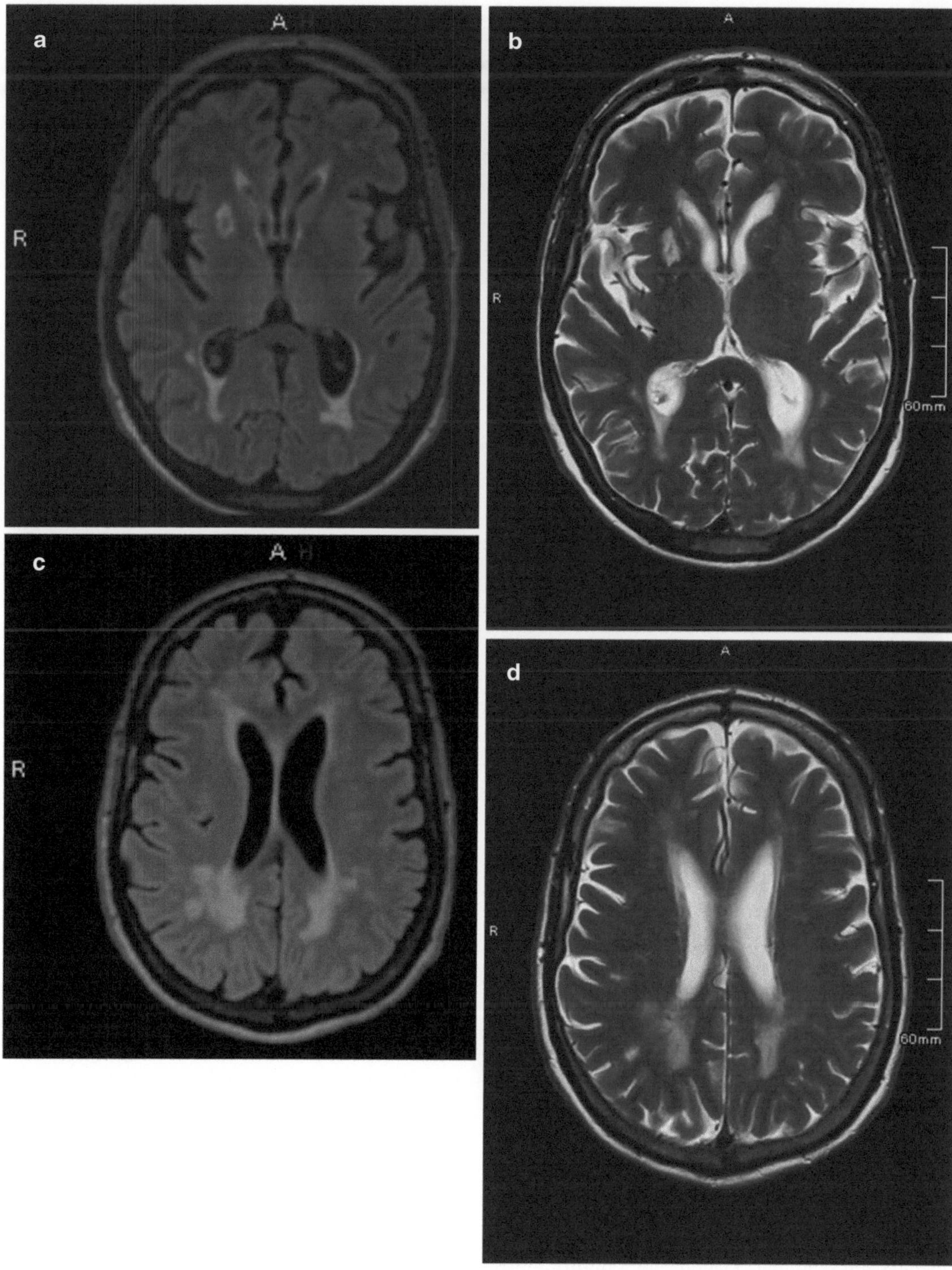


**Fig. 1** Fluid attenuated inversion recovery (FLAIR) and T2 weighted image of lacune in the anterior putamen on the right, which extended into the right caudate nucleus (**a**: FLAIR; **b**: T2) and of the confluent white matter hyperintensities which were most outspoken periventricular (**b**: FLAIR; **d**: T2). Note the lacune in the corona radiata on the right (**c**, **d**)

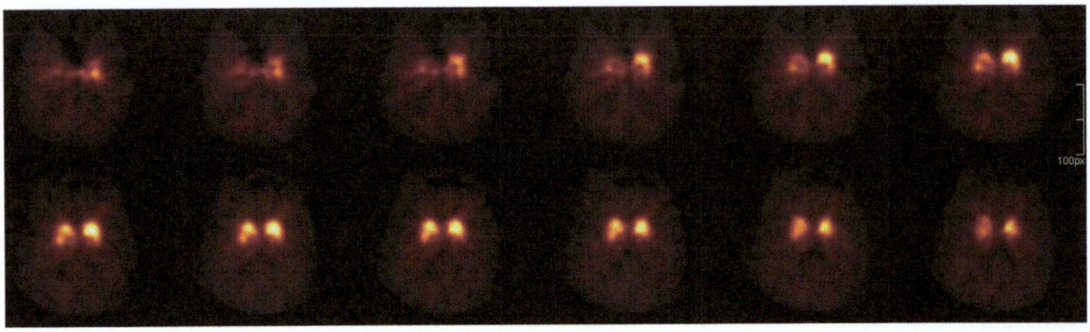


**Fig. 2** Twelve consecutive slices of the DAT SPECT scan of the striatum showing markedly reduced binding in the putamen bilaterally and focally reduced binding between the putamen and caudate nucleus on the right at the location of the lacunar infarct

## Course

After the diagnosis of probable idiopathic PD, the patient was prescribed levodopa/carbicopa 100/25 mg for 3 times a day. Initially the symptoms of the patient improved on this medication, but stabilized after a while. He experienced no side effects. The tremor of the left hand had become a less prominent symptom. Patient was referred back to his referring neurologist.

## Discussion

The presented DAT SPECT scan is rather unique in that the images show a combination of underlying nigrostriatal neurodegeneration and vascular damage (in this case lacunar infarction). The scan shows some typical characteristics of idiopathic PD. There is clearly reduced binding of the left putamen, whereas the binding in the left caudate nucleus is still largely preserved (leading to a low putamen/caudate ratio of 0.66). This is due to the pattern of nigrostriatal neurodegeneration in PD that usually starts in the posterior putamen. On the right side this pattern is not so clear due to the lacunar infarction between the caudate nucleus and putamen. Visually the binding in the left putamen is lower than on the right, as is usually the case in PD where the largest reduction is on the contralateral side of the most outspoken symptoms. The scan shows no typical pattern of vascular parkinsonism, where the striatal uptake on a DAT SPECT scan is usually preserved or mildly reduced and rather symmetric without a posterior to anterior gradient [2]. However, the lacunar infarction in the right striatum is a more strategic lesion. Combined with the quite extensive white matter disease and multiple lacunar infarctions on the MRI scan, the imaging supports mixed pathology of idiopathic PD and comorbid vascular disease.

There are three subtypes recognized for vascular parkinsonism (1) an acute or subacute onset of parkinsonism after focal infarct involving the striatal dopaminergic system; (2) insidious onset of parkinsonism predominantly affecting gait and postural instability; and (3) mixed and overlapping syndrome of neurodegenerative parkinsonism and comorbid vascular lesions which increase the parkinsonism impairment [3].

Regarding the first category, our patient indeed has a lacunar infarct in the basal ganglia, however, there is no known relationship the onset of symptoms and the occurrence of the lacunar infarct. Regarding the second category, vascular parkinsonism is usually characterized by predominant lower-body parkinsonism, postural instability, shuffling or freezing gait and absence of rest tremor [4]. Our patient has extensive subcortical white matter lesions, but his symptoms are not typical for vascular parkinsonism. There was no characteristic lower-body parkinsonism, but rather asymmetric bradykinesia and rigidity that also involved the arms (right more than left). In addition, the patient had mirror dystonia of the left hand fits with idiopathic PD, where mirror movements are typically unilateral and observed in the less affected hand during voluntary movement of the more affected hand [5]. Furthermore, the patient reported hyposmia, which is recognized as non-motor (prodromal) symptom of PD and a marker for disease severity [6]. These symptoms can therefore be attributed to underlying idiopathic PD.

Regarding the third category, it is known that the comorbid presence of vascular lesions in PD has been selectively associated with abnormal gait and balance disturbances [7]. Our patient demonstrated a stiff walking pattern and postural instability at neurological investigation. Although both can occur in the context of idiopathic PD, they might also be related to the vascular damage in this case. White matter hyperintensity burden is associated with motor and cognitive symptoms in PD patients [8] and is supposed to be a greater determinant of axial motor impairments than nigrostriatal dopaminergic neurodegeneration in PD patients with comorbid vascular disease [7].

Since nigrostriatal neurodegeneration is the primary underlying pathology in this patient, it is expected that he will respond to dopamine replacement therapy. It is important though that also vascular risk factors will be treated to limit the contribution of cerebrovascular damage to the symptoms. In this case this was taken care of by his general practitioner.

## References


1. Adriaanse SM, de Wit TC, Stam M, Verwer E, de Bruin KM, Booij J. Clinical evaluation of [$^{123}$I]FP-CIT SPECT scans on the novel brain-dedicated InSPira HD SPECT system: a head-to-head comparison. EJNMMI Res. 2018;8:4–9.
2. Zijlmans J, Evans A, Fontes F, Katzenschlager R, Gacinovic S, Lees AJ, Costa D. [$^{123}$I] FP-CIT spect study in vascular parkinsonism and Parkinson's disease. Mov Disord. 2007;22:1278–85.
3. Rektor I, Bohnen NI, Korczyn AD, Gryb V, Kumar H, Kramberger MG, de Leeuw F, Pirtošek Z, Rektorová I, Schlesinger I, Slawek J, Valkovič P, Veselý B. An updated diagnostic approach to subtype definition of vascular parkinsonism—recommendations from an expert working group. Parkinsonism Relat Disord. 2018;49:9–16.
4. Benamer HT, Grosset DG. Vascular parkinsonism: a clinical review. Eur Neurol. 2009;61:11–5.
5. Vidal JS, Derkinderen P, Vidailhet M, Thobois S, Broussolle E. Mirror movements of the non-affected hand in hemiparkinsonian patients: a reflection of ipsilateral motor overactivity? J Neurol Neurosurg Psychiatry. 2003;74:1352–3.
6. Roos DS, Twisk JWR, Raijmakers PGHM, Doty RL, Berendse HW. Hyposmia as a marker of (non-) motor disease severity in Parkinson's disease. J Neural Transm (Vienna). 2019;126:1471–8.
7. Bohnen NI, Müller ML, Zarzhevsky N, Koeppe RA, Bogan CW, Kilbourn MR, Frey KA, Albin RL. Leucoaraiosis, nigrostriatal denervation and motor symptoms in Parkinson's disease. Brain. 2011;134:2358–65.
8. Dadar M, Gee M, Shuaib A, Duchesne S, Camicioli R. Cognitive and motor correlates of grey and white matter pathology in Parkinson's disease. Neuroimage Clin. 2020;27:102353.

# Case 6: Parkinson's Disease with Left-Sided Spasticity

Elsmarieke van de Giessen

## Clinical Background

A 63-year-old man visited the neurologist for a tremor of his right hand that existed for 2 years. The tremor occurred in a specific posture, e.g., when bringing a cup to his mouth, not at rest. His left arm and leg were spastic after smallpox vaccination at infancy. There was no tremor as his left hand, but patient reported increased stiffness of the left shoulder and arm.

Furthermore, he was afraid to fall and had recently fallen from his bike. He reported hypersalivation and choking more often. There was no difficulty with eating and speaking though. According to his wife, he moved more slowly and had difficulty smiling. His smell and sleeping pattern were unchanged. There were no cognitive problems or mood disturbances.

Apart from the left-sided spasticity after smallpox vaccination, his medical history included a myocardial infarction and stenting of the right coronary artery. He used medication for cardiovascular risk factors, but no other medication. He used on average 7–10 alcoholic beverages per week, but reported no relation with the tremor. There was no family history of neurologic disorders.

A movement disorder specialist observed the following symptoms at neurologic examination. There was rigidity and a wheel cog phenomenon of the right arm, mild slowing and reduction in amplitude at finger tapping, and a postural tremor of the right hand, no rest tremor. On the left side, there was spasticity of the left arm and leg with flexion contracture of the left arm. Reflexes were normal on the right side and there was hyperreflexia and Babinski sign on the left side. There was hypesthesia left and normal sensibility on the right. Patient was bending forward while walking. He had a spastic walking pattern with circumduction of the left leg and bent left arm. Normal arm swing on the right.

There was evident salivation, suggesting hypersalivation, and central facial nerve paralysis left with hypesthesia of the left side of the face.

In summary, there was a postural tremor of the right hand, rigidity with wheel cog phenomenon of the right arm, mild bradykinesia, hypersalivation, and balance disturbances, which could all be related to possible underlying Parkinson's disease. However, neurological examination was more difficult to interpret due to spasticity of the left side of the body. Differential diagnosis was brain damage related to the event at infancy, becoming apparent later in life. Subsequently the neurologist requested an MRI scan, to assess brain damage and exclude other structural abnormalities, and a dopamine transporter single photon emission computed tomography (DAT SPECT) scan, to assess nigrostriatal neurodegeneration supporting Parkinson's disease.

E. van de Giessen (✉)
Department of Radiology and Nuclear Medicine, Amsterdam UMC, location VUmc, Amsterdam, The Netherlands



A. Varrone et al. (eds.), *Clinical Nuclear Medicine in Neurology*,
https://doi.org/10.1007/978-3-030-83598-9_6

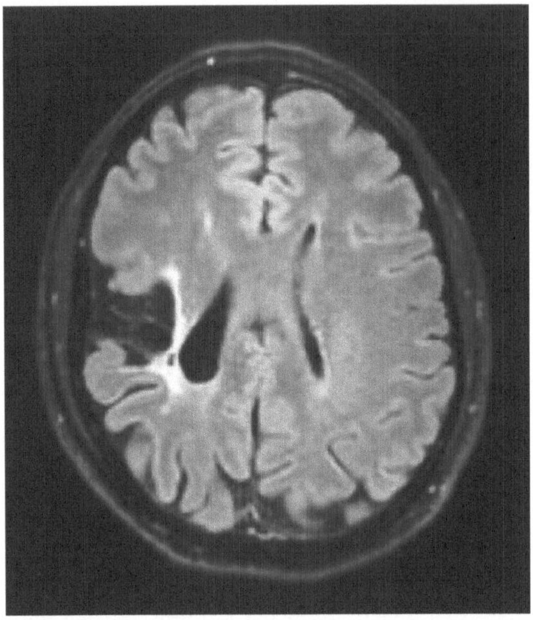

**Fig. 1** Fluid attenuated inversion recovery (FLAIR) image of frontoparietal tissue loss on the right side presumably due to stroke

## Imaging

### MRI Scan

The MRI scan showed frontoparietal tissue loss on the right side presumably as a result of stroke (Fig. 1). Otherwise there were limited vascular abnormalities with only minor white matter hyperintensities of presumed vascular origin (Fazekas score 0–1). There was no relevant atrophy. Basal ganglia, mesencephalon, and pons were normal.

### Dopamine Transporter SPECT Scan

The patient received a dopamine transporter SPECT scan of the brain according to a standard protocol that has been described in detail in Chap. 5 and previously [1]. In short, the patient was injected with 120 MBq [$^{123}$I]FP-CIT (GE Healthcare) and scanned 3 h post-injection on a brain-dedicated SPECT scanner (InSPira).

Visual was performed by an experienced reader and semiquantitative analysis was performed using BRASS (BRASS™, HERMES Medical, Sweden), as described previously [1]. The binding ratio was determined as the ratio of counts in the region of interest (caudate nucleus, putamen, whole putamen) subtracted with the counts in the reference region (occipital cortex) divided by the counts in the reference region (occipital cortex). The semiquantitative results were compared to a locally acquired database of age-matched healthy controls resulting in calculation of Z-scores.

The images showed asymmetric uptake in the striatum with reduced uptake on the left, in particular in the posterior putamen on the left (Fig. 2).

The binding ratios as determined with semiquantitative analysis were: right caudate 3.84 (Z-score 1.6), left caudate 3.65 (Z-score 1.06), right putamen 3.88 (Z-score 1.29), and left putamen 2.10 (Z-score −1.53). The putamen to caudate ratios were 1.01 for the right side and 0.58 for the left side. Although the Z-scores are considered to be within normal limits (> −2.0), the visual asymmetry and low putamen to caudate ratio on the left side are abnormal. Therefore, this scan strongly suggested nigrostriatal neurodegeneration, which given the pattern of most outspoken reduction in the posterior putamen would be consistent with Parkinson's disease.

## Conclusion

The patient presented with parkinsonian symptoms on the right side and preexisting spasticity on the left side. In combination with an abnormal DAT SPECT scan and without signs suspected for atypical parkinsonisms, he was diagnosed with probable Parkinson's disease.

## Course

The patient started taking levodopa/carbidopa 100/25 mg 3 times a day after this diagnosis. After some initial side effects (including nausea and pain

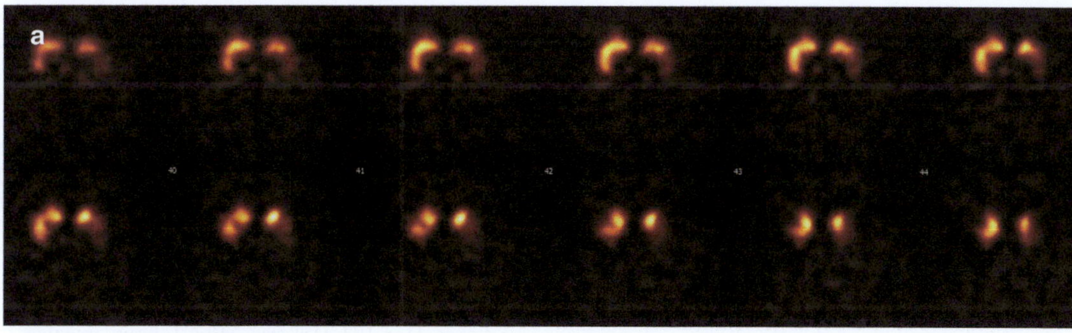


**b**

**Specific Ratio**

| Region Name | Mean | Z-Score |
|---|---|---|
| Right Caudate | 3.84 | 1.60 |
| Left Caudate | 3.65 | 1.06 |
| Right Putamen | 3.88 | 1.29 |
| Left Putamen | 2.10 | -1.53 |

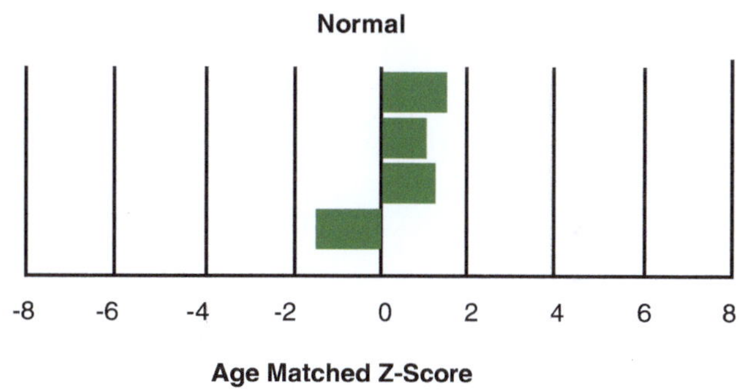


**Fig. 2** (**a**) Twelve consecutive slices of the DAT SPECT scan of the striatum showing markedly reduced binding in the putamen on the left. (**b**) Results of the semiquantitative analysis showing striatal binding ratios and *Z*-scores for the caudate nucleus and putamen for both sides

in the right leg and shoulder) without clinical response, the levodopa/carbidopa dose was increased. The side effects wore off and there was a good response with resolution of the tremor and bradykinesia 4 months after start of treatment, supporting the diagnosis of probable Parkinson's disease.

## Discussion

This case is an example of how DAT SPECT can contribute to the diagnostic process when complicated by a preexisting neurological condition. The pyramidal syndrome with left sided spasticity was clearly related to an occasion in the past in this case. However, parkinsonian symptoms may co-occur with pyramidal symptoms in rare, often inherited cases [2], complicating the diagnosis. DAT SPECT may help in these diagnostic trajectories.

Apart from the complex neurological presentation, the DAT SPECT interpretation was also not straightforward, given that the semiquantitative analysis did not show abnormal *Z*-scores compared to age- and gender-matched normal controls acquired on the same scanner. The visual asymmetry and low putamen to caudate ratio on the left side (0.58) are abnormal though. The putamen to caudate ratio can be very useful, since it is age- and camera-independent [3] and significantly lower in patients with Parkinson's disease compared to controls [4]. In general, a cutoff <0.7 to 0.8 is considered abnormal [3, 5], although there is considerable variability within patients and not all patients will meet this criterium [6].

## References


1. Adriaanse SM, de Wit TC, Stam M, Verwer E, de Bruin KM, Booij J. Clinical evaluation of [123I] FP-CIT SPECT scans on the novel brain-dedicated InSPira HD SPECT system: a head-to-head comparison. EJNMMI Res. 2018;8:4–9.
2. Tranchant C, Koob M, Anheim M. Parkinsonian-pyramidal syndromes: a systematic review. Parkinsonism Relat Disord. 2017;39:4–16.
3. Soderlund TA, Dickson JC, Prvulovich E, et al. Value of semiquantitative analysis for clinical reporting of 123I-2-beta-carbomethoxy-3beta-(4-iodophenyl)-N-(3-fluoropropyl)nortropane SPECT studies. J Nucl Med. 2013;54:714–22.
4. Seibyl JP, Marek KL, Quinlan D, et al. Decreased single-photon emission computed tomographic [123I]beta-CIT striatal uptake correlates with symptom severity in Parkinson's disease. Ann Neurol. 1995;38:589–98.
5. Varrone A, Dickson JC, Tossici-Bolt L, et al. European multicentre database of healthy controls for [123I] FP-CIT SPECT (ENC-DAT): age-related effects, gender differences and evaluation of different methods of analysis. Eur J Nucl Med Mol Imaging. 2013;40:213–27.
6. Matesan M, Gaddikeri S, Longfellow K, Miyaoka R, Elojeimy S, Elman S, Hu S, Minoshima S, Lewis D. I-123 DaTscan SPECT brain imaging in Parkinsonian syndromes: utility of the putamen-to-caudate ratio. J Neuroimaging. 2018;28:629–34.

# Case 7: Holmes Tremor

Tatiana Horowitz and Eric Guedj

## Case Summary

A 71-year-old man was initially referred for sudden left hemiparesis, hemianesthesia, anisocoria, and fourth nerve palsy. Brain MRI showed associated right thalamic and mesencephalic infarcts (Fig. 1a and 1b). He recovered rapidly after rehabilitation, and only kept slight left arm numbness. Ten months after, he developed a unilateral left rest and postural tremor, worsening with action. There were no other additional cardinal symptoms of Parkinsonism, or family history of essential tremor, or psychiatric disorder. Holmes Tremor was suspected and a [$^{123}$I]FP-CIT SPECT confirmed the diagnosis by revealing unilateral uptake amputation (Fig. 1c). Levodopa was introduced with a moderate effect on tremor.

A 71-year-old man with unilateral rest and postural tremor in postischemic context.

## Epidemiology

- Rare irregular, unilateral tremor

## Clinical Features

- Low-frequency rest and intention tremor, exacerbated by action and posture, combining nigrostriatal and cerebellar components
- Appears 4 weeks to 2 years after injury

## Pathology and Cause

- Lesion of nigrostriatal and cerebello-thalamic pathways
- Most common causes are vascular ischemic or hemorrhagic, traumatic or tumors

## Clinical Management

- Medical treatments such as levodopa or levetiracetam can be effective
- Stereotactic thalamotomy or neurostimulation of the thalamic ventral intermediate nucleus and subthalamic nucleus are proposed in severe pharmaco-resistant cases

T. Horowitz · E. Guedj (✉)
Nuclear Medicine Department, Aix Marseille Univ, APHM, CNRS, Centrale Marseille, Institut Fresnel, Timone Hospital, CERIMED, Marseille, France
e-mail: eric.guedj@univ-amu.fr



A. Varrone et al. (eds.), *Clinical Nuclear Medicine in Neurology*,
https://doi.org/10.1007/978-3-030-83598-9_7

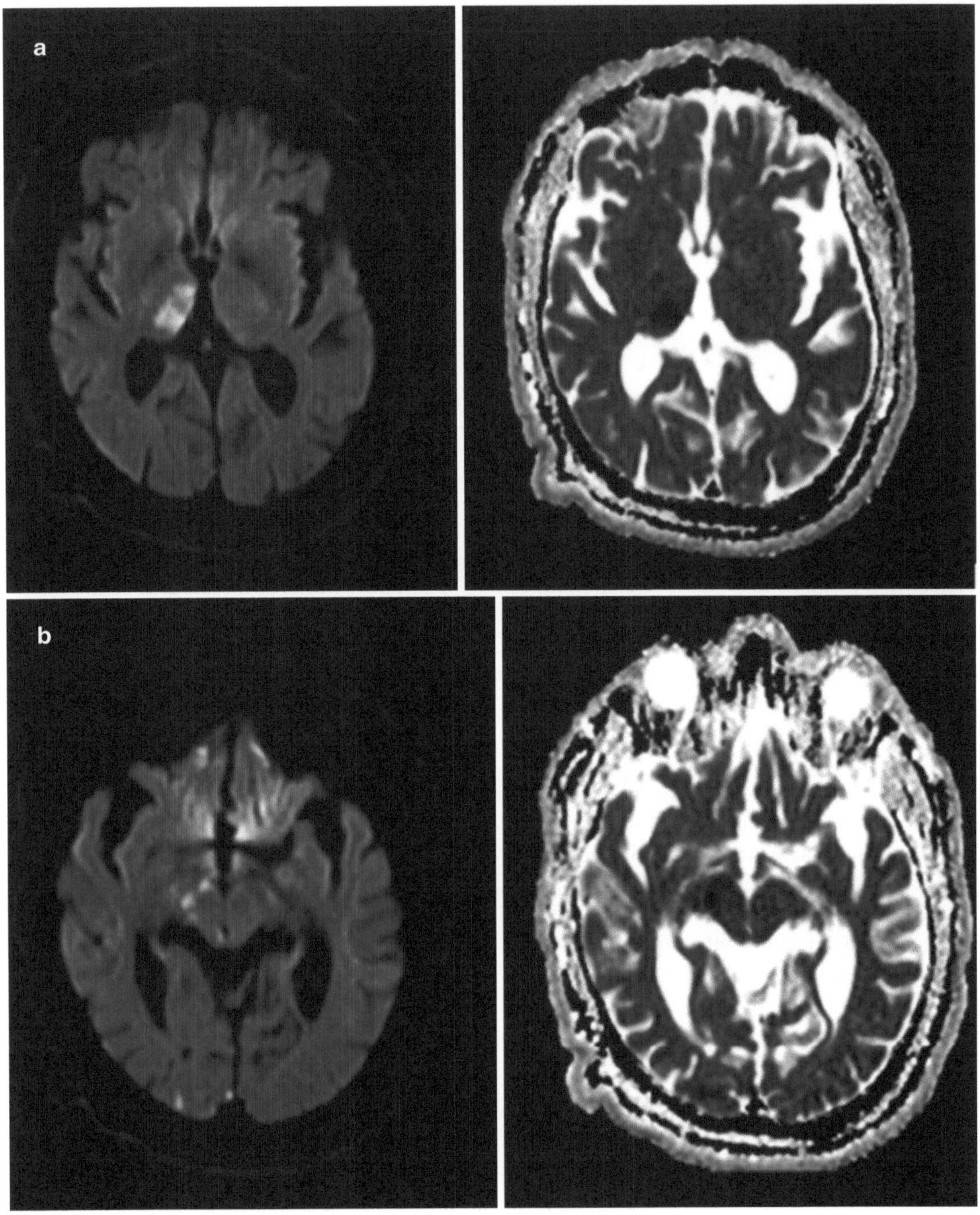


**Fig. 1** (**a**, **b**) Axial diffusion weighted MRI slice (left panels) and axial apparent diffusion coefficient MRI slice (right panels) show diffusion restriction of the right thalamus (**a**) and of the right mesencephalon (**b**) corresponding to acute ischemic strokes. (**c**) Axial [$^{123}$I]FP-CIT SPECT slices show no binding of the right caudate and putamen

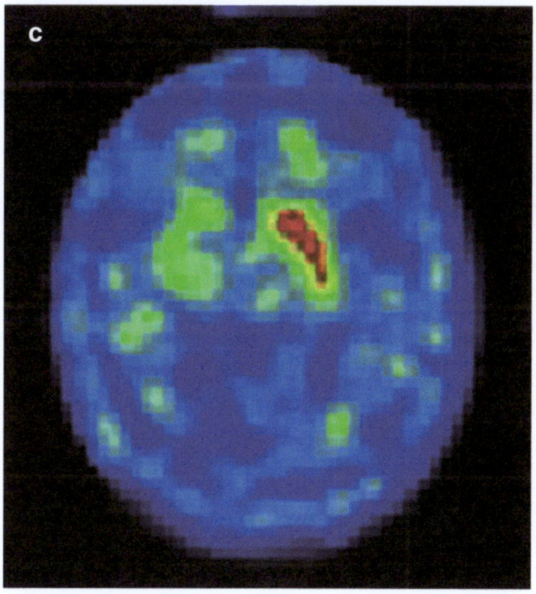


**Fig. 1** (continued)

## Imaging Findings

- MRI reveals most frequently mesencephalic or thalamic lesion
- Lesion may involve the red nucleus, globus pallidus pars interna, thalamus, cerebellum or pontomedullary junction
- [$^{123}$I]FP-CIT SPECT shows unilateral absence of basal ganglia activity

**Take-Home Message**

- Unilateral amputation of presynaptic dopaminergic uptake is suggestive of Holmes Tremor, a rare etiology of non-degenerative impaired SPECT, corresponding to a focal lesion on dopaminergic pathways.

## Further Reading

Guedj E, Witjas T, Azulay JP, de Laforte C, Peragut JC, Mundler O. Neuroimaging findings in a case of Holmes tremor. Clin Nucl Med. 2007;32(2):139–40.

Joutsa J, Shih LC, Fox MD. Mapping holmes tremor circuit using the human brain connectome. Ann Neurol. 2019;86(6):812–20.

Raina GB, Cersosimo MG, Folgar SS, Giugni JC, Calandra C, Paviolo JP, et al. Holmes tremor. Neurology. 2016;86(10):931–8.

# Case 8: Multiple System Atrophy with DAT SPECT and [$^{18}$F]FDG PET

Silvia Morbelli and Dario Arnaldi

## Background

Multiple system atrophy (MSA) is a sporadic alpha-synuclein-linked oligodendrogliopathy characterized by progressive autonomic dysfunction, cerebellar abnormalities, poorly levodopa responsive parkinsonism and corticospinal degeneration. According to the current diagnostic criteria a definite diagnosis of MSA requires the evidence of degeneration of striatonigral and olivopontocerebellar structures accompanied by glial cytoplasmic inclusions formed by fibrillized α-synuclein proteins. Conversely, criteria for probable and possible MSA both consider progressive and severe autonomic failure as the key feature, which is accompanied by a different degree of parkinsonism and cerebellar abnormalities in various combination, thus defining two categories (a) MSA with predominant parkinsonism (MSA-P) and (b) MSA with predominant cerebellar ataxia (MSA-C). It is noteworthy that such distinction, i.e., MSA-P and MSA-C, refers to the initial presentation as the predominant feature can change with time.

Clinical diagnosis may be challenging in the earliest stages when symptoms are mild and without a clear evidence of a multisystemic involvement. Indeed, in absence of parkinsonism and a clear autonomic failure, the list of differential diagnosis of cerebellar ataxia is large and includes several sporadic and hereditary disorders, such as spinocerebellar ataxias (SCAs) and Fragile X–associated tremor/ataxia syndrome (FXTAS). On the other hand, in a patient with parkinsonian features and dysautonomia, such as orthostatic hypotension and gastrointestinal dysfunction, MSA-P may be difficulty distinguished with respect to idiopathic Parkinson's disease (PD) if clinically evident ataxia is absent.

Structural and functional imaging findings can assist diagnosis and are indeed considered additional features of possible MSA in the diagnostic criteria. Indeed, typical patterns of hypometabolism in brainstem, striatum and cerebellum ([$^{18}$F] FDG PET), nigrostriatal degeneration ([$^{123}$I] FP-CIT-SPECT) and preserved cardiac post-gangliar innervation ([$^{123}$I]metaiodobenzylguanidine (MIBG) SPECT) are helpful to distinguish MSA-p or MSA-c from other conditions causing parkinsonism or cerebellar ataxia, respectively.

It should be imperative to identify MSA because of the prognosis is worse and the response to treatment is poorer compared to PD. Indeed, the worsening of motor and

S. Morbelli (✉)
IRCCS Ospedale Policlinico San Martino, Genoa, Italy

Nuclear Medicine Unit, Department of Health Sciences, University of Genoa, Genoa, Italy
e-mail: silviadaniela.morbelli@hsanmartino.it

D. Arnaldi
IRCCS Ospedale Policlinico San Martino, Genoa, Italy

Department of Neuroscience, Rehabilitation, Ophthalmology, Genetics, Maternal and Child Health (DINOGMI), University of Genoa, Genoa, Italy


A. Varrone et al. (eds.), *Clinical Nuclear Medicine in Neurology*,
https://doi.org/10.1007/978-3-030-83598-9_8

nonmotor symptoms is relentless in MSA during an average time frame of 10 years, and patients are usually bedridden in 6–8 years, with a life expectancy of 3–15 years in aggressive or more benign variants, respectively. In this context, a parkinsonian subtype is a negative prognostic factor, as well as older age at onset and early development of severe autonomic failure, whereas a cerebellar phenotype predicts slower disease progression.

## Case Presentation

- A 62-year-old Caucasian woman with no previous history of psychiatric disease or other systemic conditions other than two episodes of paroxysmal supraventricular tachycardia which have been treated with beta-blockers.
- Familiarity for Parkinson's disease (PD) for Alzheimer's disease (AD) in her maternal grandmother and paternal uncle, respectively.
- The patient complained slowness of movements, difficulties in writing and drawing, pain and rigidity in right shoulder and walking troubles with some falls without consequences in the previous months. She also reported moderate constipation, smell reduction and insomnia, mainly due to sleep behavior disorder (sudden body movements and vocalizations, like acting her dreams)
- At the neurological exam hypomimia, balance impairment and an asymmetric akinetic-rigid syndrome, mainly affecting the right limbs, without tremor, were evident (MDS-UPDRS III score = 14, Hoehn and Yahr score = 1). Mild orthostatic hypotension was also registered.
- No cognitive impairment was detected, even by means of an extended neuropsychological assessment, and blood test as well brain MRI with standard sequences were unremarkable.
- The hypothesis of PD based on the clinical presentation was confirmed by the severe nigrostriatal impairment in left putamen, detected by means of [$^{123}$I]FP-CIT-SPECT (Fig. 1).
- She was treated with dopamine-agonist (Rotigotine), MAO B inhibitor (Selegiline) and carbidopa/levodopa without any benefit on the motor syndrome.
- Given the low response to treatment, which is rather atypical in PD, she was submitted to [$^{18}$F]FDG PET which disclosed a significant hypometabolism in left putamen (Fig. 2). Such pattern of hypometabolism was consistent with atypical parkinsonism, as it differed with respect to that typically found in parieto-occipital regions in PD. The coexistence of parkinsonism with some mild dysautonomia (orthostatic hypotension, constipation) and suspected REM-behavior disorder (RBD), without any cognitive impairment, suggested an alpha-synucleinopathy.
- For the differential diagnosis between PD and MSA-P she was then further submitted to [$^{123}$I]MIBG SPECT which showed a significantly impaired cardiac autonomic innervation (Fig. 3), which was consistent with PD diagnosis.
- The patient was then periodically followed-up and treated with dopamine-agonists, MAO B inhibitors, carbidopa/levodopa and entacapone combination. Though, both orthostatic hypotension and motor impairment relentless worsened, with severe parkinsonism, dystonia of neck and right arm, dysarthria and hypophonia.
- After 2 years from the diagnosis, she needed walking assistance as the falls became frequent and she was forced into wheelchair at the last available visit (4 years since the first evaluation).
- Clinical evolution, poor response to levodopa, severe dysautonomia and [$^{18}$F]FDG PET pattern suggested the final diagnosis of MSA-P, even though [$^{123}$I]MIBG SPECT had yielded a positive result.

## Figures Legend

- **[$^{123}$I]FP-CIT-SPECT** (Fig. 1): SPECT images showing a severe dopaminergic nigrostriatal denervation in left putamen, while contralateral putamen and bilateral caudate nucleus are substantially preserved.

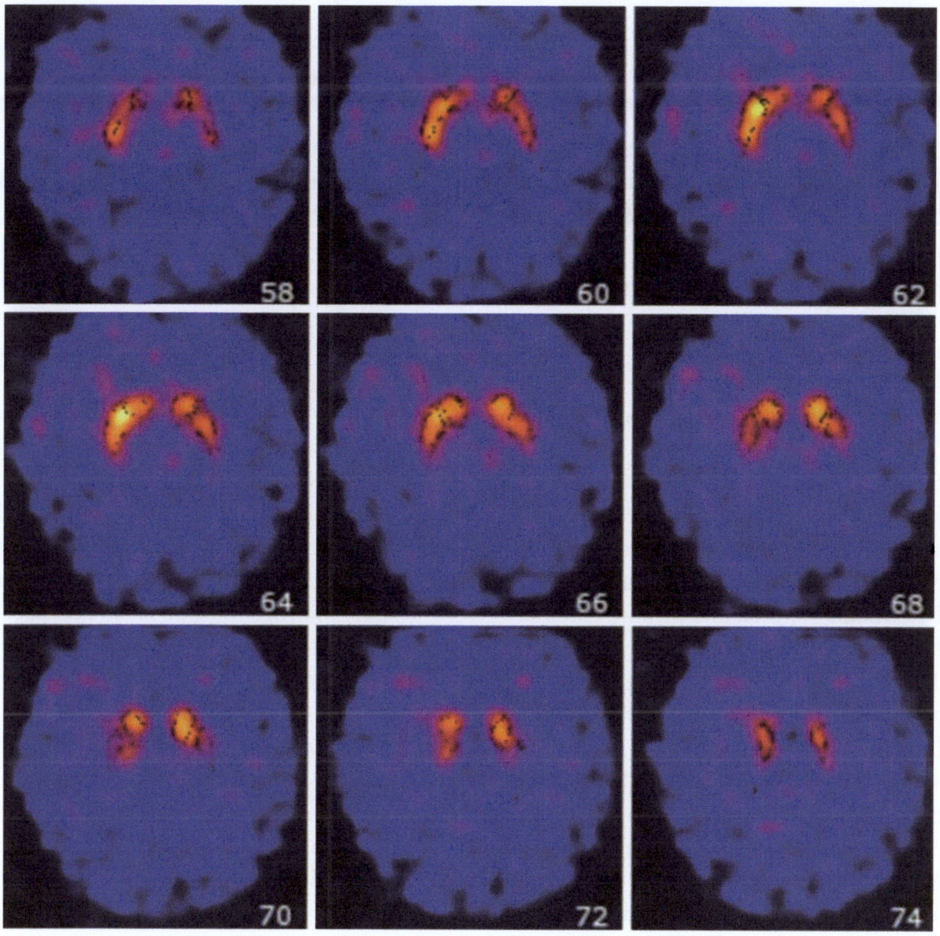


**Fig. 1** [$^{123}$I]FP-CIT-SPECT: SPECT images showing a severe dopaminergic nigrostriatal denervation in left putamen, while contralateral putamen and bilateral caudate nucleus are substantially preserved

- **[$^{18}$F]FDG PET** (Fig. 2): 18F-FDG PET images showing severe hypometabolism in left putamen (white arrow), as well as a asymmetric metabolism (left < right) in pre-rolandic frontal cortex (red arrow). No significant metabolism in brainstem, cerebellum, or other cortical areas.
- **[$^{123}$I]-MIBG SPECT** (Fig. 3): significant reduction of cardiac MIBG uptake to indicate sympathetic postganglionic myocardial denervation.

**Teaching Points**

- MSA is a sporadic alpha-synuclein-linked oligodendrogliopathy characterized by severe and progressive autonomic failure, parkinsonism, cerebellar ataxia and pyramidal signs in various combinations.
- MSA presents a major diagnostic challenge as the clinical presentation is sometimes difficultly distinguished with respect to PD or late-onset cerebellar ataxia until advanced stages of the disease.
- Structural and functional imaging findings can assist diagnosis and are indeed considered additional features of possible MSA in the diagnostic criteria.
- Putaminal, pontine, and middle cerebellar peduncle (MCP) atrophy as well as T2-signal changes including posterior putaminal hypointensity, hyperintense lateral putaminal rim, hot cross bun sign, and MCP hyperintensities are the main MRI findings which may be detected in both subtypes of MSA. Though, MRI can be unremarkable in a substantial part of patients, particularly in the earliest stages.
- [$^{18}$F]FDG PET can disclose striatal (mainly putaminal), brainstem and/or cerebellar hypometabolism, thus differentiating MSA-p and PD when parkinsonism is the main symptoms.
- The evidence of nigrostriatal dopaminergic denervation by means of [$^{123}$I]FP-CIT-SPECT is helpful to distinguish MSA-c from other causes of cerebellar ataxia. Though, a negative result does not exclude a diagnosis of MSA, especially in the very early stages of disease.
- Imaging of cardiac innervation with [$^{123}$I]MIBG SPECT can be further helpful by showing preserved sympathetic postganglionic neurons in MSA, contrary to PD.
- It has to be noted that approximately 30% of patients with MSA show decreased [$^{123}$I]MIBG uptake and confounders of [$^{123}$I]MIBG uptake such as myocardial lesions, cardiomyopathy, chronic heart failure, peripheral neuropathy or drugs must be taken into account.
- A mild degeneration of the cardiac sympathetic nerve may occur during the course of MSA, thus suggesting caution when using [$^{123}$I]MIBG in the differential diagnosis of MSA-p with PD.
- Sometimes the proper distinction between MSA-p and PD can be evident only during clinical follow-up, especially when imaging biomarkers at baseline had conflicting results.
- As long-term prognosis is worse and need of assistance is higher in patients with MSA compared to other mimicking conditions, efforts should be made to identify patients with MSA in the earliest stages for proper counseling and management.

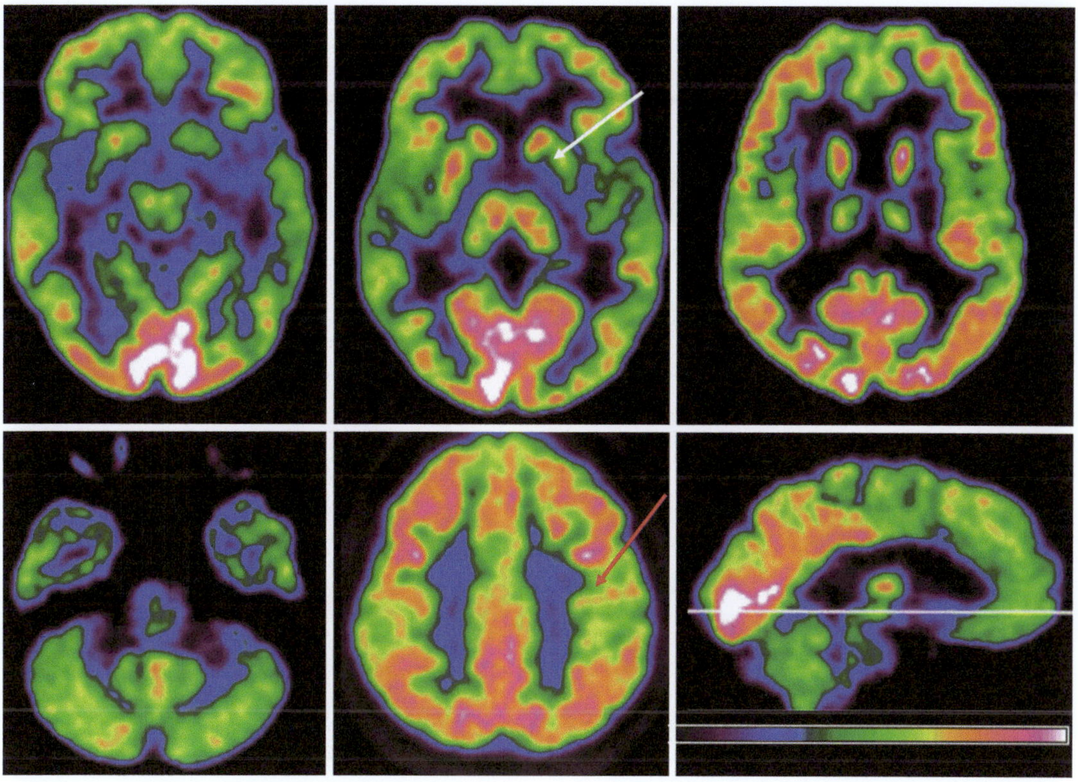

**Fig. 2** [$^{18}$F]FDG PET: [$^{18}$F]FDG PET images showing severe hypometabolism in left putamen (white arrow), as well as a asymmetric metabolism (left < right) in prerolandic frontal cortex (red arrow). No significant metabolism in brainstem, cerebellum, or other cortical areas

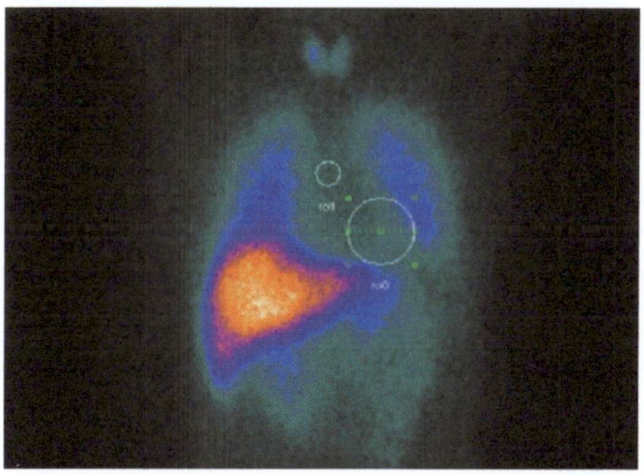

**Fig. 3** [$^{123}$I]-MIBG SPECT: significant reduction of cardiac MIBG uptake to indicate sympathetic postganglionic myocardial denervation

## Suggested Reading

Iodice V, Low DA, Vichayanrat E, Mathias CJ. Cardiovascular autonomic dysfunction in MSA and Parkinson's disease: similarities and differences. J Neurol Sci. 2011;310:133–8.

Jacobson AF, Travin MI. Impact of medications on mIBG uptake, with specific attention to the heart: comprehensive review of the literature. J Nucl Cardiol. 2015;22:980–93.

Trojanowski JQ, Revesz T, Neuropathology Working Group on MSA. Proposed neuropathological criteria for the post mortem diagnosis of multiple system atrophy. Neuropathol Appl Neurobiol. 2007;33:615–20.

# Case 9: Progressive Supranuclear Palsy: Richardson Syndrome and Parkinsonian Variants

Javier Arbizu and Gloria Martí-Andres

## Case 1 Summary

A 70-year-old, male with a with a clinical history of 1.5 years of progressive clumsiness in left hand that evolved to right hand. After a few months, he developed an additional mild dysarthria, and 2 months ago, the patient suffered an unprovoked fall. The patient had not started any treatment.

During the neurological examination it was observed a macro square wave jerks, mild dysarthria, low volume voice, akinetic-rigid syndrome asymmetric (left > right), more than two steps backward on the pull-test. The Minimental State Examination (MMSE) was 29/30, the Unified Parkinson's Disease Rating Scale part III motor examination (UPDRS-III) was 30/68, and the score in the Schwab and England Activities of Daily Living (SEADL) scale was 80% (usually completely independent).

The neuropsychological assessment showed a non-amnestic single domain mild cognitive impairment including dysexecutive syndrome (pathological Trail Making Test-part B and Luria sequence) associated with a reduced phonemic verbal fluency.

J. Arbizu (✉)
Department of Nuclear Medicine, Clinica Universidad de Navarra, University of Navarra, Pamplona, Spain
e-mail: jarbizu@unav.es

G. Martí-Andres
Department of Neurology, Clinica Universidad de Navarra, University of Navarra, Pamplona, Spain

## Images/Findings

A brain Magnetic Resonance Imaging reflected mild frontoparietal cortical atrophy, without any other pathological finding.

The [$^{18}$F]fluorodeoxyglucose Positron Emission Tomography study (FDG-PET) performed at that time (1.5 years from onset) showed a marked hypometabolism in the medial frontal and anterior cingulate cortex, while the temporoparietal cortex and primary motor cortex were preserved. Remarkably, the metabolism of the mesencephalon and partially caudates (not the putamen) was also decreased (Fig. 1). The multivariate voxel based analysis of the FDG-PET scan revealed a good matching with the PSP-related pattern (Fig. 2). The calculated PSP-RP Z-score of the FDG-PET scan performed in this case was 6.5 related to normal subjects.

The patient started treatment with levodopa (400 mg/day) but he did not show any motor improvement. During the follow-up, the patient progressively developed an oculomotor dysfunction with a vertical supranuclear gaze palsy (3 years from onset), photophobia (1.6 years), dysphagia (2 years) and the unprovoked falls were progressively more frequent. Finally, the patient died from a COVID-19 pneumonia (4.2 years from onset).


A. Varrone et al. (eds.), *Clinical Nuclear Medicine in Neurology*,
https://doi.org/10.1007/978-3-030-83598-9_9

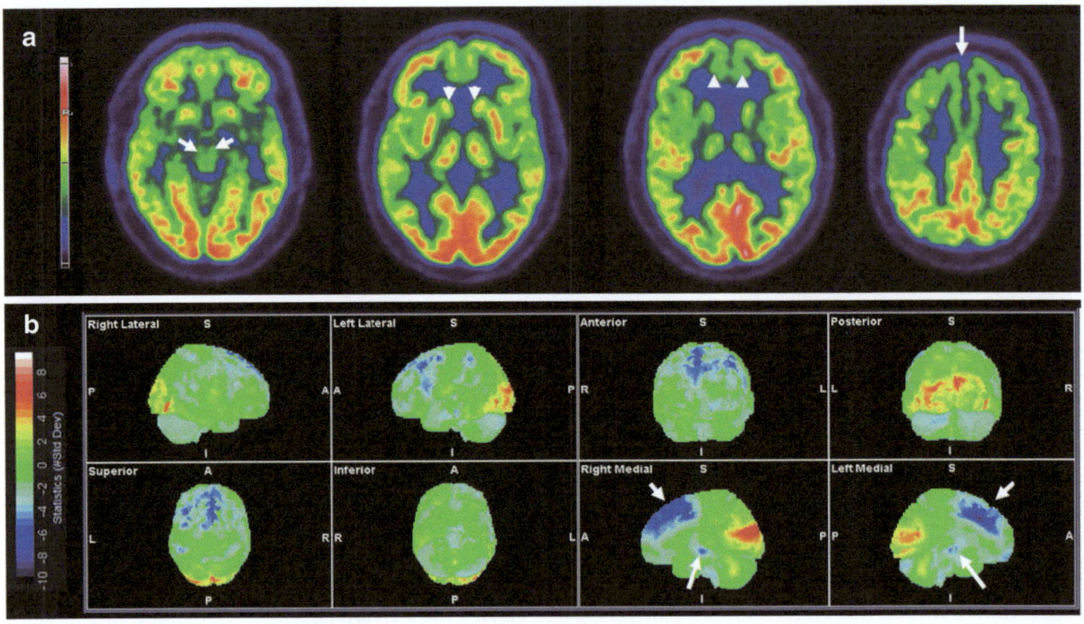


**Fig. 1** [[18]F]FDG PET scan from Case 1. (**a**) Axial slices from ventral to dorsal brain showing the characteristic areas of hypometabolism (white arrows) in the mesencephalon, caudates, dorsomedial frontal and anterior cingulate. The statistical surface projections after comparing to a normal database. (**b**) (Syngo.via Database comparison, Siemens) shows the marked hypometabolism in the medial frontal and mesencephalon (white arrows)

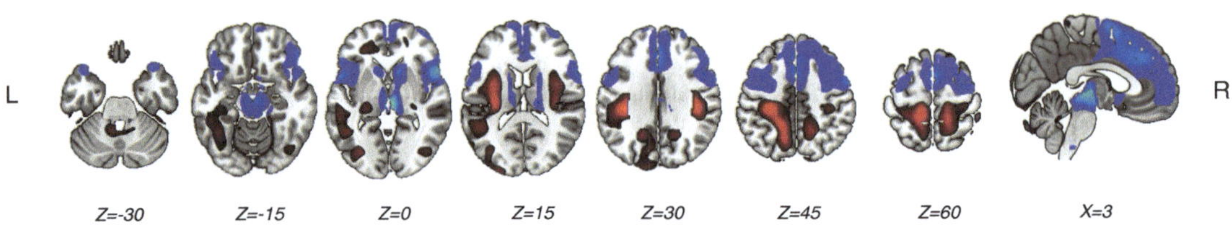


**Fig. 2** PSP-related pattern (PSP-RP) validated and cross-validated in a multicentric cohort. Axial MRI slices from ventral to dorsal brain, where areas of significant hypometabolism are superimposed in blue, and areas of hypermetabolism are in red (modified from Marti-Andres G et al. Mov Disord 2020) [1]. The calculated *Z*-score PSP-RP of the [[18]F]FDG PET scan performed in the first case was 6.5 related to normal subjects

## Diagnosis Case 1

Richardson's Syndrome subtype of Progressive supranuclear palsy.

## Case 2 Summary

An 85-year-old, male with a clinical history of 6 years of rest tremor in the right upper limb, who progressively developed generalized clumsiness and slowness of movements. Moreover, he developed a difficulty in swallowing with solid food (5 years from onset), mild constipation, and insomnia.

The neurological examination exhibited a generalized and symmetrical akinetic-rigid syndrome associated with rest tremor in upper limbs, more than two steps backward on the pull-test, and slow saccadic movement without limitation in amplitude. The MMSE was 27/30, and the UPDRS-III 20/68. The neuropsychological assessment demonstrated a multiple domain mild cognitive impairment (amnestic and dysexecutive syndromes) with pathological Luria sequence associated with a reduced phonemic verbal fluency.

## Images/Findings

The MRI excluded a vascular encephalopathy or proliferative lesions, and showed a mild symmetrical cortical and subcortical atrophy with ventricular enlargement. There were no pathological findings in the basal ganglia, mesencephalon, and substantia nigra were normal.

A presynaptic dopaminergic imaging using [$^{18}$F]Fluorodopa PET study was prescribed to elucidate the suspected neurodegenerative origin of this parkinsonian syndrome. The study showed a bilateral nigrostriatal dopaminergic denervation (right hemisphere more affected) involving both putamen and caudates but with rostro-caudal gradient (Fig. 3). The striatal to occipital ratio on the right putamen was 1.99 and 2.17 on the left putamen (both >2 SD compared to normal database; DopaSoft PMOD), and the ratio on the caudates were 1.81 on the right side and 1.91 on the left (both >2 SD; DopaSoft PMOD).

The patient started with Levodopa 200 mg/8 h. However, there was no or at least mild response to L-dopa (UPDRS-III 15, 25% reduction). In the following months, he developed unprovoked falls and a decreased speed (6.5 years from onset). The MMSE was 28/30, and the UPDRS-III and SEADL fell to 22/68 and 50%, respectively.

At that time, a FDG-PET scan was performed to evaluate the neuronal activity pattern (6.5 years from onset) in an attempt to clarify the differential diagnosis with non-responder parkinsonism. The FDG-PET images reflected an extensive and marked hypometabolism of the frontal lobe (dorsolateral and dorsomedial cortex) as well as anterior cingulate (Fig. 4), particularly on the right hemisphere where the parietal cortex was also involved. Additionally, the activity in both caudates, mesencephalon and thalamus was notably decreased, predominantly on the right side. We calculated the expression of the previously defined PSP-related pattern (PSP-RP) [1] at individual level using a multivariate analysis (Scaled Subprofile Modeling/Topographic Profile Rating) by applying an automated algorithm written in-house, based on the method described by Spetsieris and Eidelberg and detailed elsewhere [2]. The PSP-RP *Z*-score in this case was 9.42 related to normal subjects (see [1] for software analysis details).

During the next 6 months, the patient developed an oculomotor dysfunction with a reduction in amplitude of vertical greater than horizontal saccadic eye movements (7 years from onset).

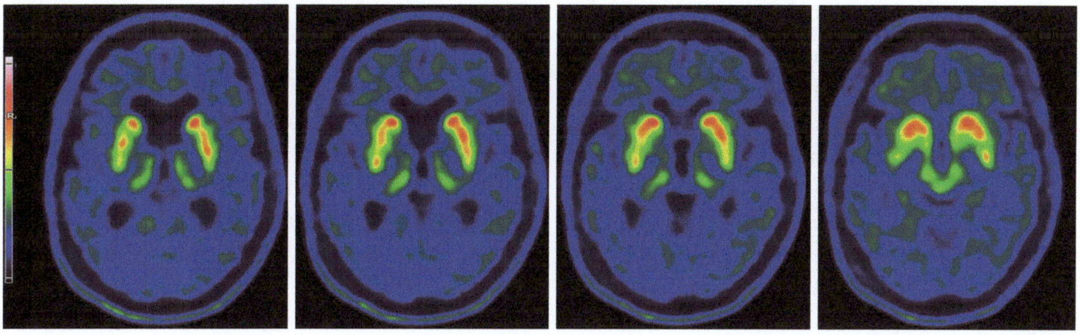

**Fig. 3** [$^{18}$F]Fluorodopa PET scan of Case 2. Sequential axial images showing a decrease of the striatal presynaptic dopaminergic activity predominantly on the right hemisphere, and with some rostro-caudal gradient

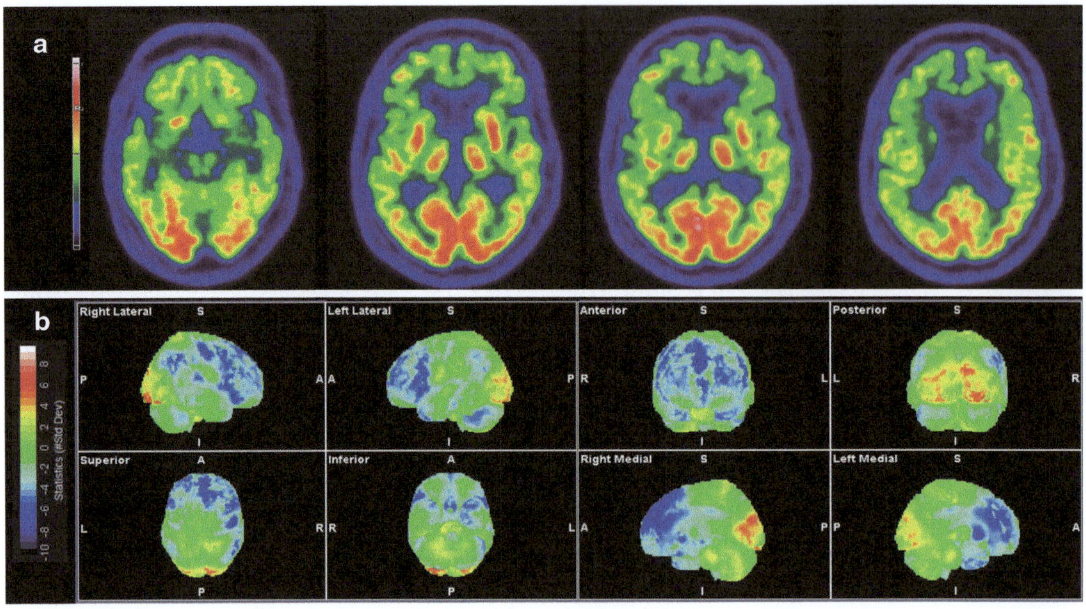


**Fig. 4** [18F]FDG PET scan performed in Case 2. Axial slices (**a**) show a marked and extensive hypometabolism in the frontal cortex including dorsolateral, medial frontal and frontoinsular regions, and subcortical involvement in the mesencephalon, caudates. These findings can be easily seen in the statistical surface projections after comparing to a normal database (**b**) (Syngo.via Database comparison, Siemens)

## Diagnosis Case 2

Parkinsonian subtype of progressive supranuclear palsy.

## Discussion

Progressive supranuclear palsy (PSP) is a primary tauopathy associated with a heterogeneous spectrum of clinical features, including a variable combination of behavioral, cognitive (language and executive dysfunction) and motor phenomena (ocular motor dysfunction, postural instability, and Parkinsonism) [3–6].

The International Parkinson and Movement Disorder Society developed criteria for the diagnosis of PSP (MDS-PSP) define different clinical subtypes of PSP [7].

Richardson's syndrome (PSP-RS), or classical subtype, is the most frequent clinical presentation of PSP and it is characterized by gait instability and falls in the first 3 years, oculomotor dysfunction (hypokinetic, hypometric saccades vertical more so than horizontal, vertical supranuclear gaze palsy), pseudobulbar signs and cognitive impairment (executive dysfunction, personality changes, apathy). This PSP subtype has an average survival of only 5–7 years [8].

Parkinsonian variant of PSP is the second most frequent subtype of PSP (PSP-P). These patients present an asymmetric parkinsonian syndrome, rest tremor and in some cases an initial and transitory response to levodopa. Over time, these patients may develop gait disturbances and oculomotor dysfunction. This PSP subtype has an average survival of 9–10 years from disease onset [9].

PSP-RS patients show atrophy of the midbrain and superior cerebellar peduncles as the disease progresses. Many midbrain-based MRI morphometric measures have shown good sensitivity and specificity for differentiating PSP-RS from other parkinsonian disorders, such as the mid-sagittal midbrain area, the pons area to midbrain area ratio (P/M) and the Magnetic Resonance Parkinsonism Index (MRPI). However, their sensitivity is not good enough for early stages of the disease [10], neither display an adequate diagnostic performance in differentiating among atypical PSP subtypes nor subtypes from Parkinson's disease (PD) patients [11].

FDG-PET has shown to be a useful diagnostic tool for differentiating PSP-RS and PSP-P subtypes from PD patients and healthy controls, even at early stages of the disease [1]. The FDG-PET pattern is characterized by a relative hypometabolism in the midbrain, basal ganglia, thalamus and frontoinsular cortices and a relative hypermetabolism in the cerebellum, primary sensorimotor and posterior insula cortices. Moreover, each variant shows its particular differences [1]. PSP-RS showed the largest cortex involvement with a relative hypometabolism in frontoinsular cortex and relative hypermetabolism in parieto-occipital cortex. Parkinsonian variant shows an additional asymmetrical involvement of anterior putamen.

The first case presented here shows the role of FDG-PET as supportive diagnostic tool for an early diagnosis of a classic PSP-RS subtype. In this case, the patient showed only mild clinical signs of postural instability and oculomotor dysfunction which reach only a diagnostic certainty level of suggestive of PSP. Moreover, the patient had not received any dopaminergic treatment to assess the clinical response. However, the FDG-PET performed at 1.5 years from the onset of the disease showed a clear increased expression of the PSP-related pattern, which supported the final clinical diagnosis of PSP obtained after the clinical follow-up.

The second case is a representative of PSP-P subtype. The diagnosis of these patients is challenging as they show an initial clinical course indistinguishable from PD patients (rest tremor, asymmetric parkinsonism). However, during follow-up develop atypical signs (late-onset postural instability, oculomotor dysfunction and/or cognitive deficits) and differ in clinical management response and prognosis. In this case, the FDG-PET shows a marked expression of PSP-RP which was greater than in Case 1 (*Z*-score 9.4 vs. 6.5) and probably related to the larger disease duration (6.5 years vs. 1.5 years from onset). These findings supported the final clinical diagnosis of PSP-P subtype.

## Conclusions

Molecular imaging biomarkers can help clinicians to reach an etiological diagnosis of parkinsonian syndromes. While presynaptic dopaminergic imaging supports the neurodegenerative origin of parkinsonism, the differential diagnosis between PD and atypical syndromes like PSP or multiple system atrophy can be elucidated by means of FDG-PET. FDG-PET has shown common brain metabolic abnormalities within different PSP subtypes, that can be used as a diagnostic tool for differentiating PSP from PD patients and healthy controls, even at early stages of the disease [1].

## References


1. Martí-Andrés G, Bommel L, Meles SK, et al. Multicenter validation of metabolic abnormalities related to PSP according to the MDS-PSP criteria. Mov Disord. 2020;35(11):2009–18.
2. Meles SK, Renken RJ, Pagani M, et al. Abnormal pattern of brain glucose metabolism in Parkinson's disease: replication in three European cohorts. Eur J Nucl Med Mol Imaging. 2020;47(2):437–50.
3. Respondek G, Stamelou M, Kurz C, et al. The phenotypic spectrum of progressive supranuclear palsy: a retrospective multicenter study of 100 definite cases. Mov Disord. 2014;29:1758–66.
4. Respondek G, Kurz C, Arzberger T, et al. Which ante mortem clinical features predict progressive supranuclear palsy pathology? Mov Disord. 2017;32(7):995–1005. https://doi.org/10.1002/mds.27034.
5. Williams DR, de Silva R, Paviour DC, et al. Characteristics of two distinct clinical phenotypes in pathologically proven progressive supranuclear palsy: Richardson's syndrome and PSP-parkinsonism. Brain. 2005;128:1247–58.
6. Williams DR, Holton JL, Strand C, et al. Pathological tau burden and distribution distinguishes progressive supranuclear palsy-parkinsonism from Richardson's syndrome. Brain. 2007;130:1566–76.
7. Höglinger GU, Respondek G, Stamelou M, et al. Clinical diagnosis of progressive supranuclear palsy:

the movement disorder society criteria. Mov Disord. 2017;32:853–64.
8. Ali F, Josephs K. The diagnosis of progressive supranuclear palsy: current opinions and challenges. Expert Rev Neurother. 2018;18(7):603–16. https://doi.org/10.1080/14737175.2018.1489241.
9. Dell'Aquila C, Zoccolella S, Cardinali V, et al. Predictors of survival in a series of clinically diagnosed progressive supranuclear palsy patients. Parkinsonism Relat Disord. 2013;19:980–5.
10. Whitwell JL, Höglinger GU, Antonini A, et al. Radiological biomarkers for diagnosis in PSP: where are we and where do we need to be? Mov Disord. 2017;32:955–71.
11. Picillo M, Tepedino MF, Abate F, et al. Midbrain MRI assessments in progressive supranuclear palsy subtypes. J Neurol Neurosurg Psychiatry. 2020;91:98–103.

# Case 10: Progressive Supranuclear Palsy (PSP)

Silvia Morbelli and Maria Isabella Donegani

## Introduction

Progressive supranuclear palsy (PSP) is a late-onset neurodegenerative tauopathy characterized by the intra-cerebral aggregation of the microtubule-associated tau protein. It is associated to both neuronal and glial lesions in the basal ganglia, diencephalon, brainstem and cerebellum, with involvement of the neocortex relatively variable on an individual patient basis.

The prevalence of PSP is 5.8–6.5 per 100.000, the average age at symptoms onset is around mid-60 and survival from onset averages 7 years with a wide variance. The cause is yet mostly unknown.

Clinically, it is characterized by a wide variety of signs and symptoms that makes correct diagnosis commonly delayed after symptom onset, even up to 3–4 years.

Most common initial symptoms include movement and gait disorders (gait ignition failure and freezing of gait), and severe postural instability that leads to early unprovoked falls (mostly backwards). Eyes movement disorders are extremely characteristic and mainly concern voluntary eye movements and the inability to make vertical saccades. This restriction of the range of vertical gaze can lead in the advanced disease to a vertical supranuclear gaze palsy.

Behavioural features can include apathy, executive dysfunction, emotional lability, compulsive behaviour and inappropriate sexual behaviour.

Many patients with PSP have dementia or cognitive impairment that can include executive and inhibition deficits and memory impairment (poor episodic memory and visuospatial functions).

In the late stages, swallowing difficulties, severe dysphonia and dysarthria, emotional lability, inspiratory sighs, stereotyped moaning or groaning can occur.

Based on the different clinical presentations, different subtypes of PSP have been identified. Richardson's syndrome (PSP-RS) is the most frequent phenotype, comprising of 50% or more of PSP cases with postmortem confirmation. PSP-parkinsonism (PSP-P) and PSP with progressive gait freezing (PSP-PGF) have a more benign course. PSP-P and PSP-PGF are sometimes referred as the 'brain stem' variants of PSP, as opposed to the 'cortical' variants, which present with predominant cortical features including PSP-corticobasal syndrome (PSP-CBS), PSP-behavioural variant of frontotemporal dementia (PSP-bvFTD) and PSP-progressive non-fluent aphasia (PSP-PNFA).

Early clinical diagnosis of PSP is challenging but relevant for prognostic reasons. In particular, the differential diagnosis between PSP and

S. Morbelli (✉) · M. I. Donegani
IRCCS Ospedale Policlinico San Martino, Genoa, Italy

Nuclear Medicine Unit, Department of Health Sciences, University of Genoa, Genoa, Italy
e-mail: silviadaniela.morbelli@hsanmartino.it



A. Varrone et al. (eds.), *Clinical Nuclear Medicine in Neurology*,
https://doi.org/10.1007/978-3-030-83598-9_10

Parkinson disease (PD) might be particularly complex, especially in case of PSP-P in which features of PD, such as asymmetrical tremor, bradykinesia, and rigidity, overlap with the clinical presentation of PSP. Moreover, in PSP patients a possible initial misleading positive response to Levodopa treatment can be present.

## Case Presentation

- A 70-year-old woman, 8 years education, right-handed.
- In the last 2 years postural instability with frequent falls. She also complains of dysphagia.
- At the neurological examination, the patient presented vertical gaze palsy, postural instability, rigidity and bradykinesia.
- Neuropsychological tests were performed resulting in a mild dementia, with MMSE = 23 and CDR = 1.0. Activities of daily living were mildly impaired. Objective neuropsychological deficit on attention and executive functions was found.
- MRI was reported as negative for any relevant findings.
- Considered the presence of mild dementia (with more prominent executive dysfunction) and the hypokinetic-rigid parkinsonian syndrome, the patient was submitted to [$^{18}$F]FDG PET/CT to evaluate patterns of hypometabolism for the differential diagnosis within neurodegenerative parkinsonian syndromes.

## Imaging Findings

Brain [$^{18}$F]FDG PET revealed a bilateral hypo metabolism in the anterior cingulate gyrus and a mild asymmetry (left < right) in fronto-insular cortex and frontal dorsolateral cortex. In addition, the uptake in the basal ganglia (especially in the putamen) seems to be only mildly bilaterally reduced (Fig. 1).

- To better explore the underlying pattern of hypometabolism in the [$^{18}$F]FDG PET images a semiquantitative evaluation with a voxel-based software was performed (Fig. 2).
- Hypometabolism in frontal cortex and anterior cingulate was confirmed. A significant hypometabolism in both putamen was also clearly confirmed with respect to normal controls. Moreover, the semiquantitative analysis allowed to identify the presence of hypometabolism in the brain stem.
- Those finding, which the visual evaluation alone could not fully appreciate, correspond precisely to the pattern of hypometabolism of PSP as described in the literature (cfr. Booij et al. QJNM 2012)

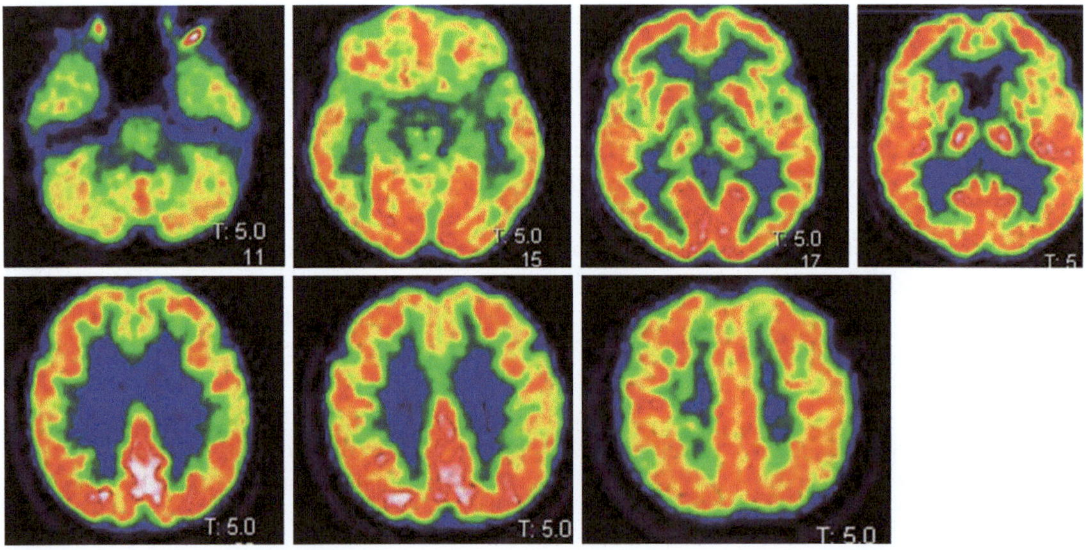


**Fig. 1** Axial brain [$^{18}$F]FDG-PET images

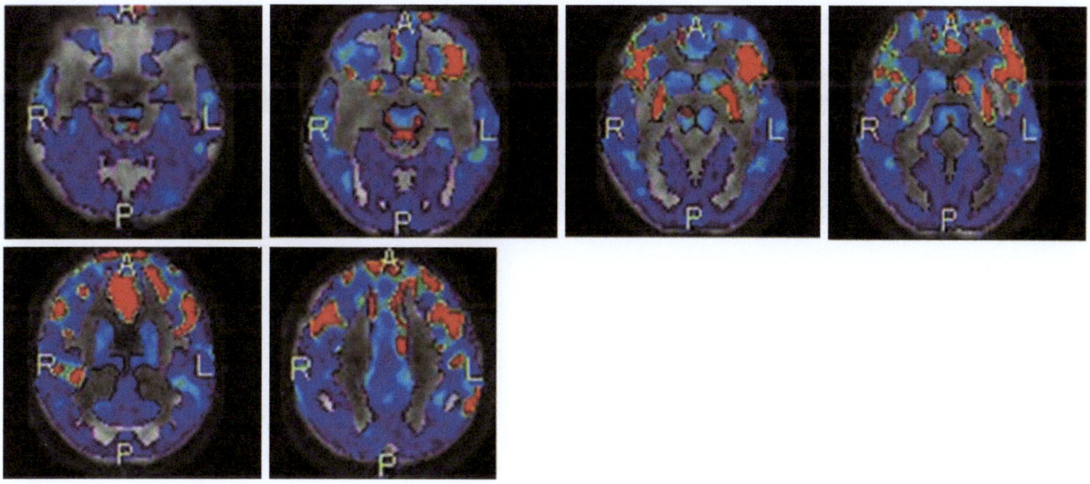


**Fig. 2** Voxel-based analysis. The areas of significant hypometabolism with respect to age-matched controls are labelled in red

**Take Home Messages**

- [$^{18}$F]FDG PET can be useful for the differential diagnosis within neurodegenerative parkinsonian syndrome (especially when an atypical parkinsonism is suspected). In fact each neurodegenerative parkinsonian syndrome is characterized by a peculiar pattern of hypometabolism.
- Hypometabolism in subcortical and/or medial structures is less easily detected by visual analysis. Indeed when mild to moderate hypometabolism involves bilaterally subcortical structures (close to the median line), semiquantitative voxel-based analysis and comparison with normal subjects' database might be of help for the identification of the hypometabolic pattern. This approach might thus be particularly useful for to fully exploit the value of [$^{18}$F]FDG PET in the framework of atypical parkinsonian syndromes (which differently from idiopathic Parkinson Disease) are expected to involve basal ganglia and other subcortical regions. In this case the confirmation of the involvement of bilateral putaminal nuclei and the identification of brain stem hypometabolism allow to support the presence of PSP.
- Of note, in the present study, the MRI was reported as normal. Indeed, given the key role of midbrain in PSP-related pathological process, a number of specific MRI morphometric measures have been proposed. In particular the hummingbird sign reflecting midbrain atrophy, has previously been shown to separate patients with progressive PSP from those with PD. However the lack of reported alteration on MRI in presence of hypometabolism on [$^{18}$F]FDG PET is not surprising as the hummingbird sign (such as other MRI signs in patients with atypical parkinsonian syndromes) tends to suffer from low sensitivity, especially in early disease stages.

## Suggested Reading

Booij J, Teune LK, Verberne HJ. The role of molecular imaging in the differential diagnosis of parkinsonism. Q J Nucl Med Mol Imaging. 2012;56:17–26.

Dickson DW, Ahmed Z, Algom AA, Tsuboi Y, Josephs KA. Neuropathology of variants of progressive supranuclear palsy. Curr Opin Neurol. 2010;23:394–400.

Ling H. Clinical approach to progressive supranuclear palsy. J Mov Disord. 2016;9:3–13.

Walker Z, Gandolfo F, Orini S, Garibotto V, Agosta F, Arbizu J, et al. Clinical utility of FDG PET in Parkinson's disease and atypical parkinsonism associated with dementia. Eur J Nucl Med Mol Imaging. 2018;45:1534–45.

# Case 11: Corticobasal Syndrome: [$^{18}$F]FDG and Amyloid PET

Javier Arbizu and Gloria Martí-Andres

## Case Summary

A 65-year-old female with a 3 years history of difficulties in dressing, self-care neglecting, and memory loss. She additionally developed clumsiness and slowness in the left limbs. Progressively, she showed spatial orientation problems and became afraid of getting lost in case of going out alone. She felt sad with a tendency to cry. Her husband described some behavioral changes with a progressive apathy and anhedonia, and sometimes she showed socially inappropriate behaviors.

The neurological examination exhibited bradypsychia, positive applause sign, ideatory apraxia associated with a mild bradykinesia in the left hand, mild rigidity in neck, hyperreflexia in the left limbs, and short-stepping gait with a reduction of left arm swing.

The neuropsychological assessment showed a multiple domain non-amnestic mild cognitive impairment (dysexecutive syndrome and visuospatial dysfunction). The patients scored 25/30 in the Mini Mental State Examination (MMSE) and 21 in the geriatric depression scale (severe depressive).

J. Arbizu (✉)
Department of Nuclear Medicine, Clinica Universidad de Navarra, University of Navarra, Pamplona, Spain
e-mail: jarbizu@unav.es

G. Martí-Andres
Department of Neurology, Clinica Universidad de Navarra, University of Navarra, Pamplona, Spain

## Imaging/Findings

The magnetic resonance imaging (MRI) ruled out any vascular or tumoral lesion in the brain and showed a generalized cortical atrophy with predominance in frontoparietal lobes slightly more marked in the right side.

In order to elucidate the possible etiology of this syndrome, a brain positron emission tomography (PET/CT) with [$^{18}$F]FDG (FDG-PET), and an amyloid PET/CT using [$^{18}$F]Florbetapir (amyloid PET) were performed (3 years from onset). The FDG-PET (Fig. 1) exhibited a markedly asymmetric metabolism due to a right hemisphere hypometabolism of the dorsolateral frontal and parietal cortex with mild anterior temporal engagement. Moreover, the motor and premotor cortices were also involved in the hypometabolic areas. However, the metabolism of the posterior cingulate was well preserved. At the subcortical level, there was a clearly asymmetric hypometabolism in the right putamen, concerning particularly the posterior part. In the amyloid PET (Fig. 2), the radiotracer uptake was limited to the white matter and the frontal, parietal, posterior cingulate and temporal cortices were unaffected. Consequently, this study was negative for the presence of Alzheimer pathology in the brain.


A. Varrone et al. (eds.), *Clinical Nuclear Medicine in Neurology*,
https://doi.org/10.1007/978-3-030-83598-9_11

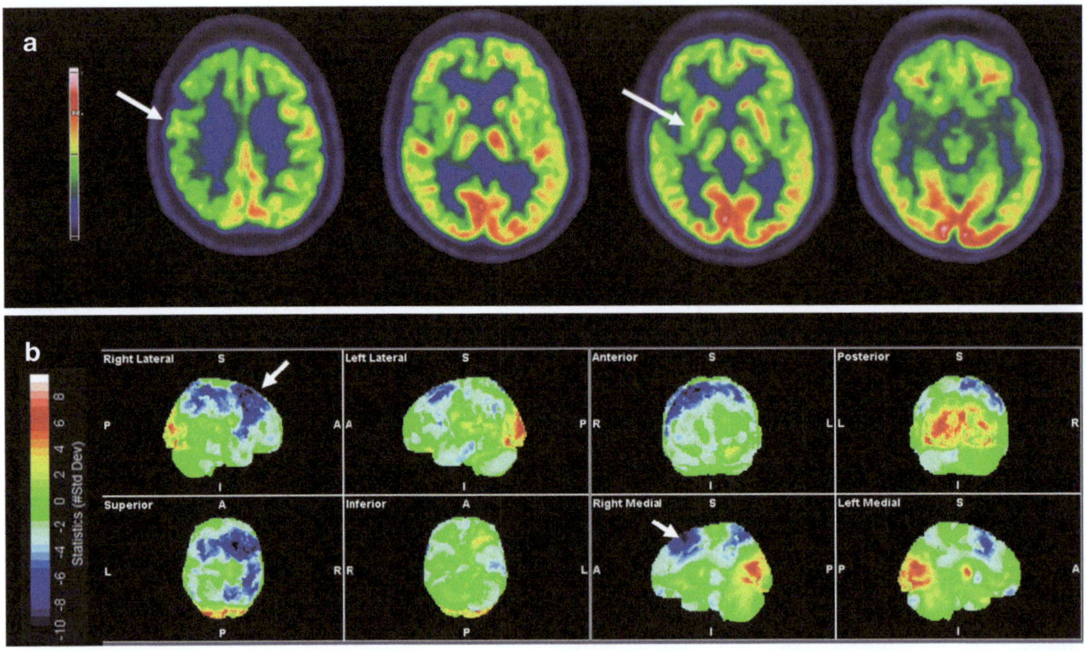


**Fig. 1** [18F]FDG-PET scan. (**a**) Sequential axial slices showing hypometabolism of the right frontoparietal cortex including premotor cortex (short white arrow), and right posterior putamen (long white arrow). (**b**) Three-dimensional stereotactic surface projections maps (3D-SSP, Syngo.via database comparison, Siemens), showing cortical areas with significant hypometabolism (>2 SD) are shown in dark blue. Interestingly, the motor cortex in the right hemisphere is affected (long white arrow) as well as sensorimotor cortex in the medial projections (short white arrow)

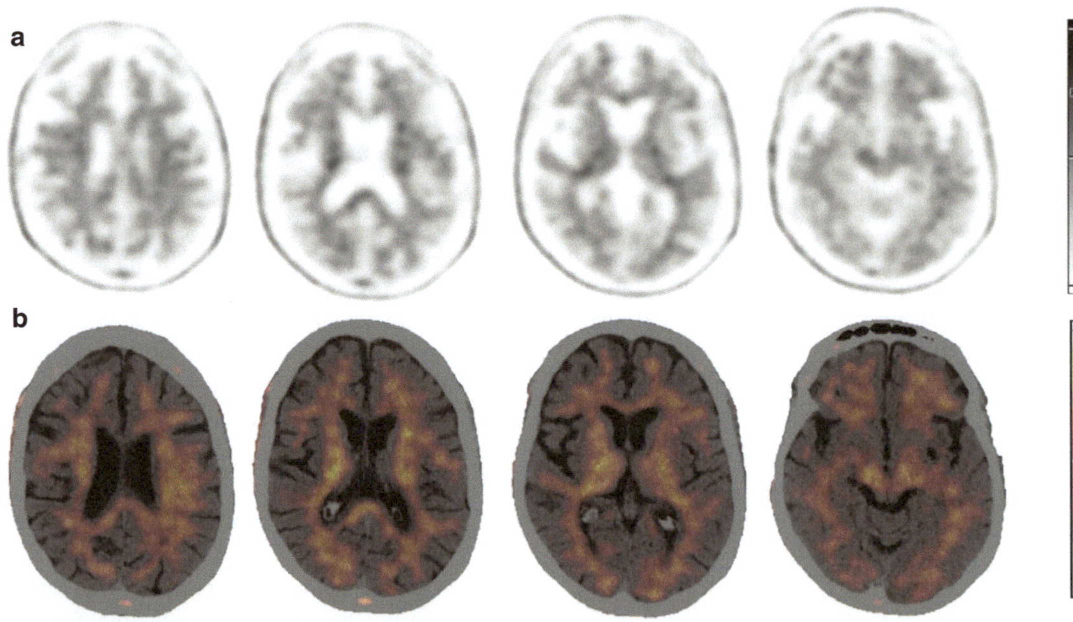


**Fig. 2** Negative amyloid PET/CT using [18F]Florbetapir. Sequential axial PET images (**a**) and fused PET and CT images (**b**) showing a high activity in the with matter tracts without any increase in the frontal, temporal, parietal, and posterior cingulate cortex

During the follow-up, the patient presented a progressive impairment of both, cognitive (dementia) and motor features. She developed a constructive apraxia, emotional lability, disinhibition with compulsive eating behavior, echolalia, an alien limb, and a worsening of the asymmetrical rigid-akinetic syndrome (4 years from onset). In the last years of the disease, she developed a language impairment, decreased velocity of vertical saccades, and a dystonia in her left hand (5–6 years from onset).

## Diagnosis

Probable cortibasal syndrome due to corticobasal degeneration.

## Discussion

The current diagnostic criteria propose a list of clinical phenotypes associated with the pathology of corticobasal degeneration (CBD) [1]. A probable corticobasal syndrome (CBS) is included among them, and it is defined as an asymmetric presentation of 2 of: (a) limb rigidity or akinesia, (b) limb dystonia, (c) limb myoclonus plus 2 of: (d) orobuccal or limb apraxia, (e) cortical sensory deficit, (f) alien limb phenomena (more than simple levitation). CBD is the most common cause of CBS, and it accounts for almost 50% of all CBS cases. Progressive supranuclear palsy (PSP) and Alzheimer's disease (AD) pathologies follow CBD as the second and third most common causes [2]. Clinical criteria for CBD validation studies found that approximately 50% of false positive cases had AD, so it is presumed that the exclusion of amyloid biomarkers would have improved the specificity of the diagnosis (e.g., cerebrospinal fluid or imaging biomarkers).

It is well known that patterns of atrophy in CBS vary according to pathologic diagnosis. Widespread atrophy points toward a pathologic diagnosis of frontotemporal lobe degeneration associated to transactive response DNA binding protein of 43 kDa (FTLD-TDP) or AD, with frontotemporal loss suggesting FTLD-TDP and temporoparietal loss suggesting AD. On the contrary, more focal atrophy predominantly involving the premotor and supplemental motor area suggests an underlying tauopathy (CBD or PSP) [3].

Moreover, FDG-PET studies in CBS patients due to CBD show an asymmetric hypometabolism in the lateral premotor cortex, supplementary motor area, motor cortex, prefrontal lobes, superior parietal lobes, striatum, and thalamus. Compared to PSP-Richardson's Syndrome patients, CBS patients due to CBD usually show a more severe and widespread cortical hypometabolism, with greater involvement of the parietal lobes and less involvement of the midbrain [2]. Interestingly, cortical hypometabolism in CBD patients usually appears earlier than presynaptic dopaminergic deficit because of delayed neuronal loss in the substantia nigra [4].

The prevalence of amyloid PET positivity in CBS decreased with age [5], thus AD is more likely to be the causative pathology in young CBS patients, whereas a primary tauopathy becomes more likely with increasing age. CBS patients that are amyloid positive on PET tend to show greater visuospatial deficits, a higher rate of sentence repetition impairment, more functional decline and greater atrophy in the posterior temporal lobe compared to amyloid negative patients [6].

## Conclusions

CBS can be a common phenotype of different neurodegenerative conditions such as CBD, AD, and PSP among others. This case illustrates a CBS that combined a frontoparietal cognitive dysfunction with an asymmetrical parkinsonism in which the etiological diagnosis remained uncertain. In the presence of a generalized cortical atrophy, FDG-PET showed an asymmetrical corticobasal hypometabolism suggestive of CBS due to CBD, and the absence of beta-amyloid deposition on PET scanning ruled out AD. Thus, the imaging biomarkers helped the clinician to reach a most probable clinical diagnosis of CBS secondary to a tauopathy, probably due to CBD, at early stages.

## References

1. Armstrong MJ, Litvan I, Lang AE, Bak TH, Bhatia KP, Borroni B, et al. Criteria for the diagnosis of corticobasal degeneration. Neurology. 2013;80:496–503.
2. Saranza GM, Whitwell JL, Kovacs GG, Lang AE. Corticobasal degeneration. In: Brain mapping. Amsterdam: Elsevier; 2019. p. 87–136.
3. Whitwell JL, Jack CR Jr, Parisi JE, Senjem ML, Knopman DS, Boeve BF, et al. Imaging correlates of pathology in corticobasal syndrome. Neurology. 2010;75:1879–87.
4. Pirker S, Perju-Dumbrava L, Kovacs GG, Traub-Weidinger T, Pirker W. Progressive dopamine transporter binding loss in autopsy-confirmed corticobasal degeneration. J Parkinsons Dis. 2015;5(4):907–12.
5. Ossenkoppele R, Jansen WJ, Rabinovici GD, Knol DL, van der Flier WM, van Berckel BN, et al. Prevalence of amyloid PET positivity in dementia syndromes. JAMA. 2015;313:1939.
6. Burrell JR, Hornberger M, Villemagne VL, Rowe CC, Hodges JR. Clinical profile of PiB-positive corticobasal syndrome. PLoS One. 2013;8:e61025. https://doi.org/10.1371/journal.pone.0061025.

# Case 12: Huntington's Disease with Atypical Onset

Silvia Morbelli and Giulia Ferrarazzo

## Introduction

Huntington's disease (HD) is an inherited neurodegenerative disorder caused by an expanded CAG repeat in the HTT gene, resulting in loss of GABAergic medium spiny neurons in the striatum and in cortical areas.

A clinical diagnosis is typically made in presence of involuntary movement (often in patients with family history of disease). Patients may experience progressive cognitive decline, and many exhibit behavioral and psychiatric symptoms. Irritability, depression, obsessive and compulsive symptoms, apathy and psychosis occur at rates higher than seen in the non-HD population.

Cognitive or psychiatric symptoms may also be present before motor symptoms accordingly, HD represents a rare but important differential diagnosis of cognitive impairment. Other clinical features of HD are discussed in the chapter discussing the case of "Huntington's Disease with Psychiatric Onset."

Genetic testing represents current routine standard in the diagnostic pathway of HD. However patients might be submitted to [$^{18}$F]FDG PET to support the differential diagnosis of cognitive impairment or behavioral disturbances and nuclear medicine physician should be aware of the peculiar features of FDG PET in these patients to guide images interpretation and suggest subsequent diagnostic work-up.

S. Morbelli (✉) · G. Ferrarazzo
IRCCS Ospedale Policlinico San Martino, Genoa, Italy

Nuclear Medicine Unit, Department of Health Sciences, University of Genoa, Genoa, Italy
e-mail: silviadaniela.morbelli@hsanmartino.it

## Case Presentation

- A 42-year-old man with no previous history of psychiatric disease or symptoms.
- Father affected by early onset dementia occurring from the age of 50 (suspected FTD).
- Mother described as "depressed" never referred to a neurological or psychiatric evaluation.
- 12 years of schooling (Degree in business administration).
- Regular sleep-wake rhythm (his wife refers that he kicks when he sleeps).

## Clinical Presentation and Past Clinical History

- His wife reports marked distractibility and slowdown in daily actions, although she also reports he has always been shy and clumsy in movements.
- He reports two episodes of "convulsive syncope."



A. Varrone et al. (eds.), *Clinical Nuclear Medicine in Neurology*,
https://doi.org/10.1007/978-3-030-83598-9_12

- He was referred to neurological visits 1 year before (namely after the second episode of "convulsive syncope" → the neurologist reported depression symptoms, psychomotor slowdown with apathy).

## Neurological Evaluation

Neurological examination was substantially normal except for tiny fidgety movements of both arms.

Activities of daily living: 6/6. Instrumental activities of daily living: 6/8.

Electroencephalography: normal findings.

Neuropsychological assessment: borderline score for memory tests and abnormal score for verbal and categorial fluency.

## Imaging Evaluation

Due to claustrophobia the patient refused to perform brain MRI scan and was referred to brain FDG PET/CT to exclude a neurodegenerative disease (namely, frontotemporal dementia, given familiar history):

FDG PET/CT findings:

- Coregistered CT showed mild degree of atrophy (more than what expected given patient's age). Atrophy was more evident in temporolateral cortex at CT (Fig. 1)
- Marked bilateral hypometabolism in basal ganglia (yellow arrows in Fig. 2) and in temporolateral and posterior parietal cortex (red and blue arrows in Fig. 2).

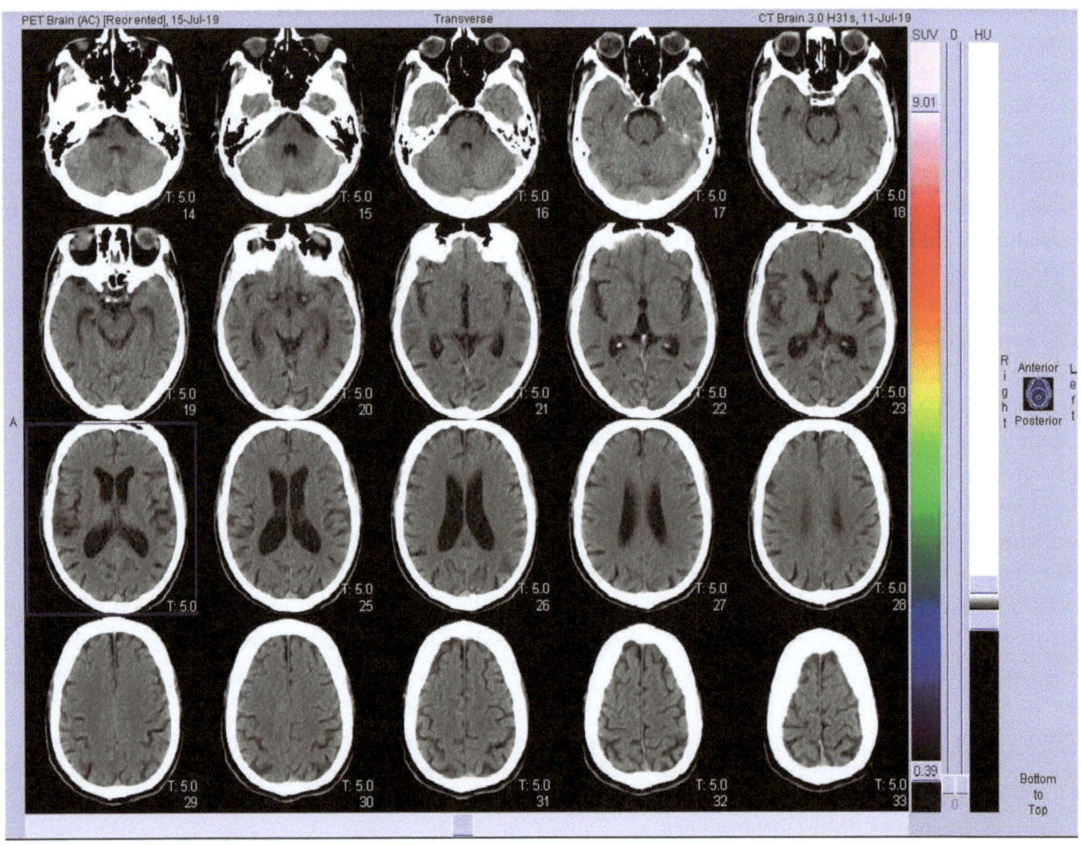


**Fig. 1** Axial brain TC images

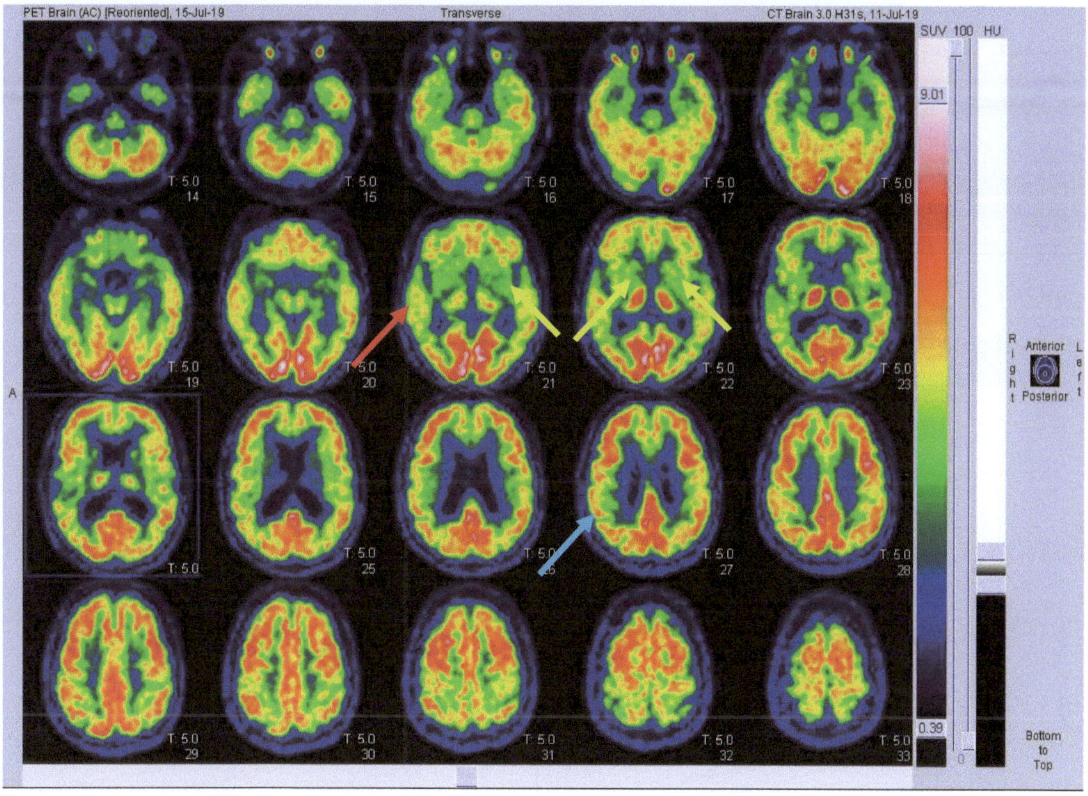


**Fig. 2** Axial brain FDG PET images

Given the peculiar presentation and the FDG PET findings, the patient underwent also DAT SPECT that showed marked reduced uptake in both putamen and left caudatus (Fig. 3).

Imaging findings showing marked bilateral hypometabolism in basal ganglia associate with nigrostriatal dopaminergic deficit may, at least in theory, lead to differential diagnosis between:

- atypical parkinsonisms (MSA, PSP, CBD)
- accumulation diseases (Brain Iron Accumulation, Wilson's disease)
- chorea syndromes (Huntington's Disease, McLeod Syndrome).

In the present case, given the differential diagnosis between accumulation diseases and chorea syndromes.

Laboratory tests: cupraemia and ceruloplasmin resulted slightly reduced (not significant).

Peripheral blood smear: acanthocytes evaluation (negative).

Genetic test revealed gene IT15 mutation, confirming HD diagnosis.

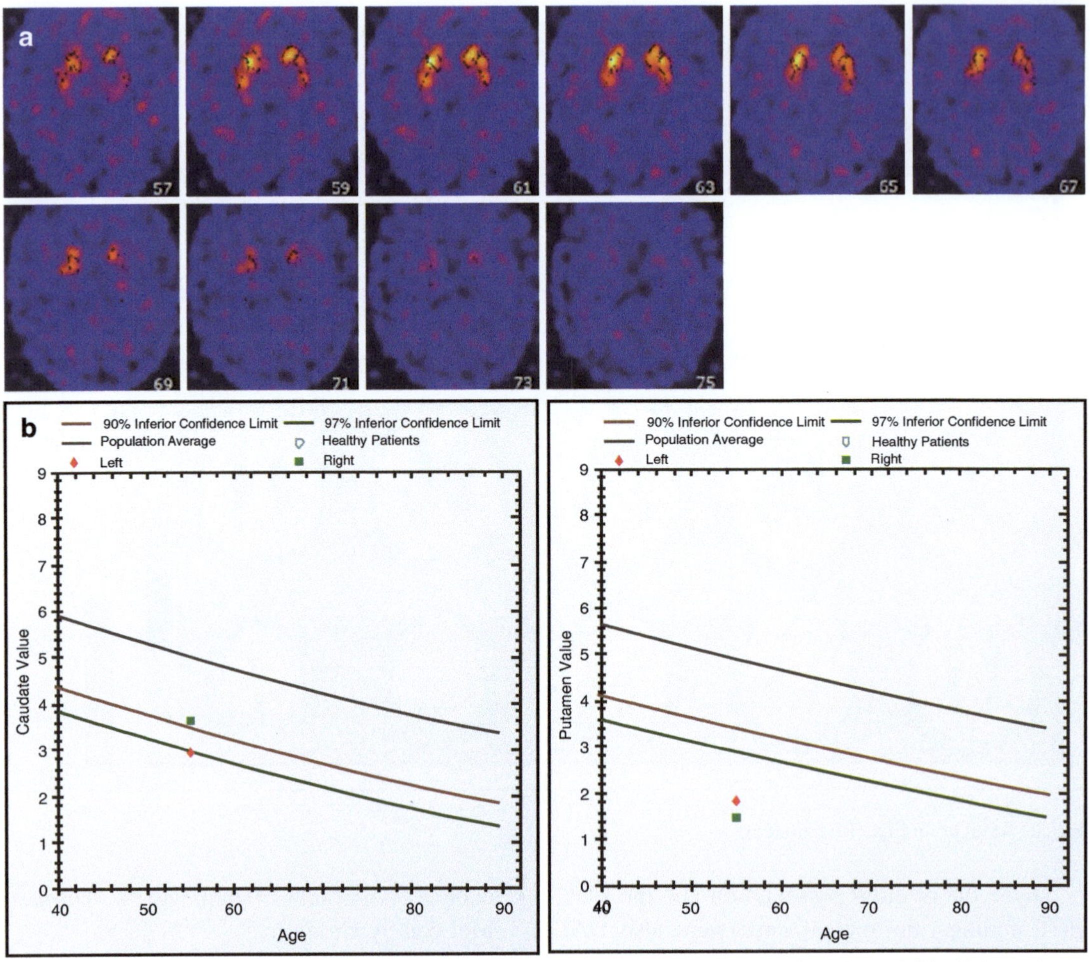


Caudate: patient activity (left side in red, right side in green)

Putamen: patient activity (left side in red, right side in green)

**Fig. 3** Axial brain DAT SPECT images (**a**) and semiquantification results (**b**) showing reduced uptake with respect to age-matched controls using basal ganglia software (BasGan V2)

**Take Home Messages**

- [$^{18}$F]FDG PET can reveal unexpected findings (marked hypometabolism in the basal ganglia) and guide subsequent diagnostic work-up in patients with behavioral symptoms in whom the differential diagnosis is needed between neurodegenerative diseases (in this case due to HD but more often possibly due to frontotemporal dementia) and psychiatric disorders.
- The pathological process of Huntington's disease (HD) preferentially targets spiny neurons in the striatum, with later involvement of the substantia nigra. However, [$^{123}$I]FP-CIT SPECT can be altered in several patients especially in patients with relatively more advanced disease. [$^{123}$I]FP-CIT SPECT could also be useful in investigating the progression of presynaptic dopaminergic degeneration in HD, possibly acting as a disease biomarker, providing an objective method for measuring the effectiveness of future neuroprotective therapies.

## Suggested Reading

Ellis N, Tee A, McAllister B, Massey T, McLauchlan D, Stone T, et al. Genetic risk underlying psychiatric and cognitive symptoms in Huntington's disease. Biol Psychiatry. 2020;87:857–65.

Gamez J, Lorenzo-Bosquet C, Cuberas-Borrós G, Carmona F, Badía M, Castilló J, Badía M, de Fabregues O, Hernández-Vara J, Castell-Conesa J. Progressive presynaptic dopaminergic deterioration in Huntington disease: a [123I]-FP-CIT SPECT two-year follow-up study. Clin Nucl Med. 2014;39(3):e227–8. https://doi.org/10.1097/RLU.0b013e31828162cd. PMID: 23531734

Genetic Modifiers of Huntington's Disease (GeM-HD) Consortium. Identification of genetic factors that modify clinical onset of Huntington's disease. Cell. 2015;162:516–26.

Gusella JF, MacDonald ME, Lee JM. Genetic modifiers of Huntington's disease. Mov Disord. 2014;29:1359–65.

Hwang WJ, Yao WJ. SPECT study of the nigrostriatal dopaminergic system in Huntington's disease. J Neuroimaging. 2013;23(2):192–6. https://doi.org/10.1111/j.1552-6569.2011.00671.x. PMID: 22211920

# Case 13: Huntington's Disease with Psychiatric Onset

Silvia Morbelli and Matteo Bauckneht

## Introduction

Chorea is a hyperkinetic movement syndrome characterized by brief, involuntary, and random muscle contractions. Chorea is defined as being "primary" when it is attributed to Huntington's disease (HD) or to other genetic etiologies, while it is defined as "secondary" when it is related to infectious, pharmacologic, metabolic, autoimmune disorders, or paraneoplastic syndromes.

HD is the autosomal dominant monogenic neurodegenerative disease, with a prevalence of 0.4–5.7 per 100.000 worldwide. It is caused by an expanded CAG trinucleotide repeat sequence in the huntingtin gene on chromosome 4, resulting in loss of GABAergic medium spiny neurons in the striatum and in cortical areas.

Besides motor symptoms, at the earlier stages HD can be, less frequently, characterized by cognitive symptoms (slowed mentation, attention, mental flexibility, planning and emotion recognition) as well as psychiatric symptoms (depression, apathy, impulsivity, irritability, disinhibition, and psychosis).

Genetic testing is the current routine standard in the diagnostic pathway of HD. FDG-PET is usually not performed in patients with suspected HD. However, HD represents a rare but important differential diagnosis of cognitive impairment, especially when cognitive or psychiatric symptoms are the initial signs of the disease, before motor symptoms are manifest. In these cases, FDG-PET images interpretation may play a central role in the differential diagnosis by guiding the diagnostic hypothesis and the subsequent diagnostic flow-chart.

## Case Presentation

- A 56-year-old Caucasian man with no previous personal history or family history of neuropsychiatric disease.
- After his mother's death, the patient developed anxiety and depressive mood. He sought medical attention for conciliation insomnia, hyperoxia, emotional liability, anxiety, and obsessive-compulsive symptoms.
- He was treated with Sodium Valproate 300 mg and Paroxetine 20 mg, without a measurable response.
- After a multidisciplinary discussion, aiming to disclose the eventual organic nature of the obsessive-compulsive disorder (i.e., underlying neurodegenerative etiology, namely in the spectrum of frontotemporal degeneration), the patient was referred to neuropsychological tests, brain MRI and brain FDG-PET.

S. Morbelli (✉) · M. Bauckneht
IRCCS Ospedale Policlinico San Martino, Genoa, Italy

Nuclear Medicine Unit, Department of Health Sciences, University of Genoa, Genoa, Italy
e-mail: silviadaniela.morbelli@hsanmartino.it


A. Varrone et al. (eds.), *Clinical Nuclear Medicine in Neurology*,
https://doi.org/10.1007/978-3-030-83598-9_13

- The neuropsychological assessment resulted negative, apart from the occurrence of non-perseverative errors at the Wisconsin card sorting test (WCST), and MRI was reported as negative for brain atrophy or any other relevant findings (Fig. 1).
- Similarly, FDG-PET excluded the occurrence of FTD. However, it unexpectedly revealed a severe bilateral striatal hypometabolism (yellow arrows in Fig. 2). Mild hypometabolism involving the right temporal lobe was also observed (red arrow in Fig. 2).
- The patient was referred thus to the Neurology Department. During this examination, the patient was alert and oriented to person, place, and time. His temperature, heart rate, blood pressure, respiratory rate, blood oxygen level, and blood work results were normal. The neurological examination revealed the occurrence of mild hyperkinetic motor signs and nonspecific upper limb weakness without movement difficulties.
- The psychiatric symptoms of the patient, in addition to the FDG-PET findings, and the hyperkinetic motor signs, were in favor of the diagnosis of HD. Genetic test revealed 41 triplets on one Huntingtin allele, confirming the diagnosis.

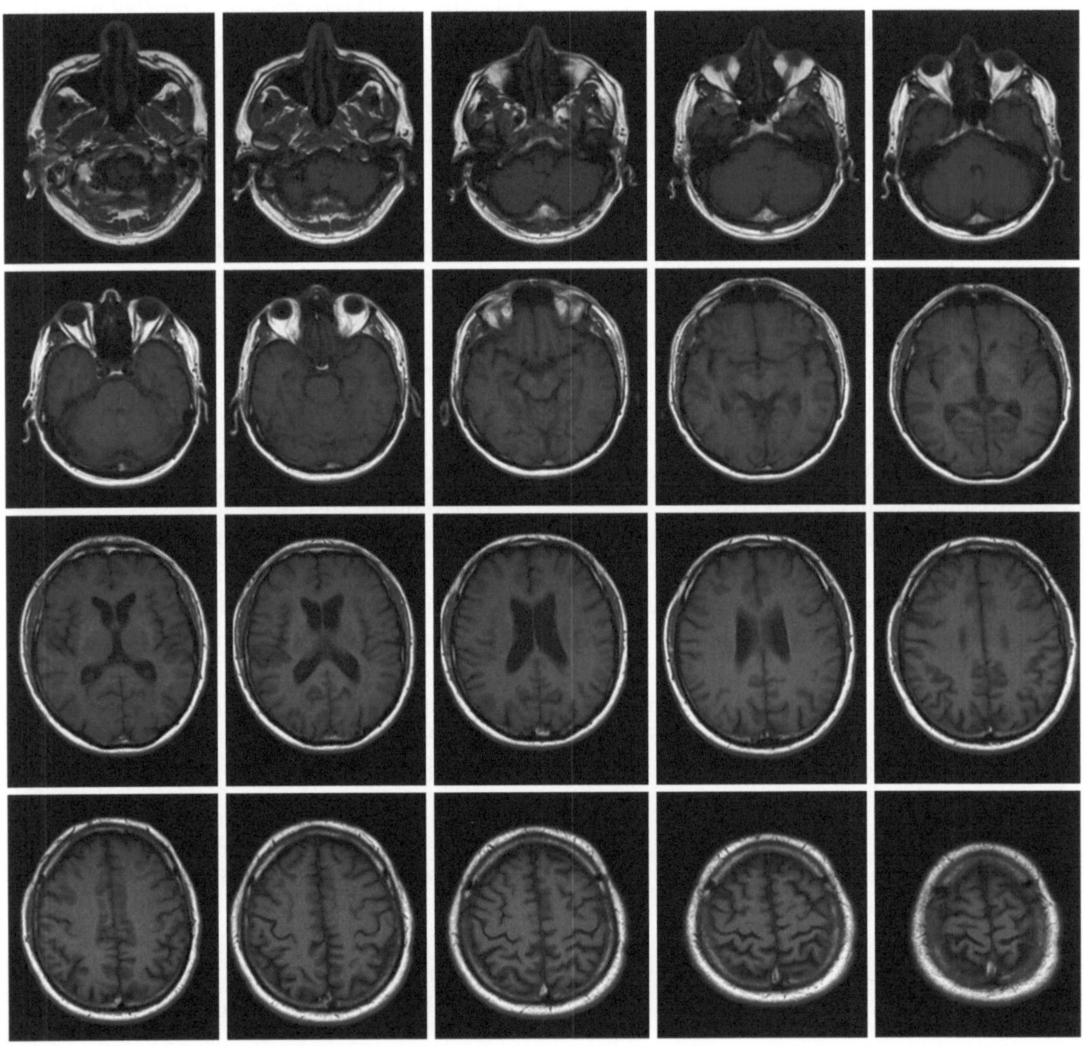

**Fig. 1** Axial T1-weighted MRI images

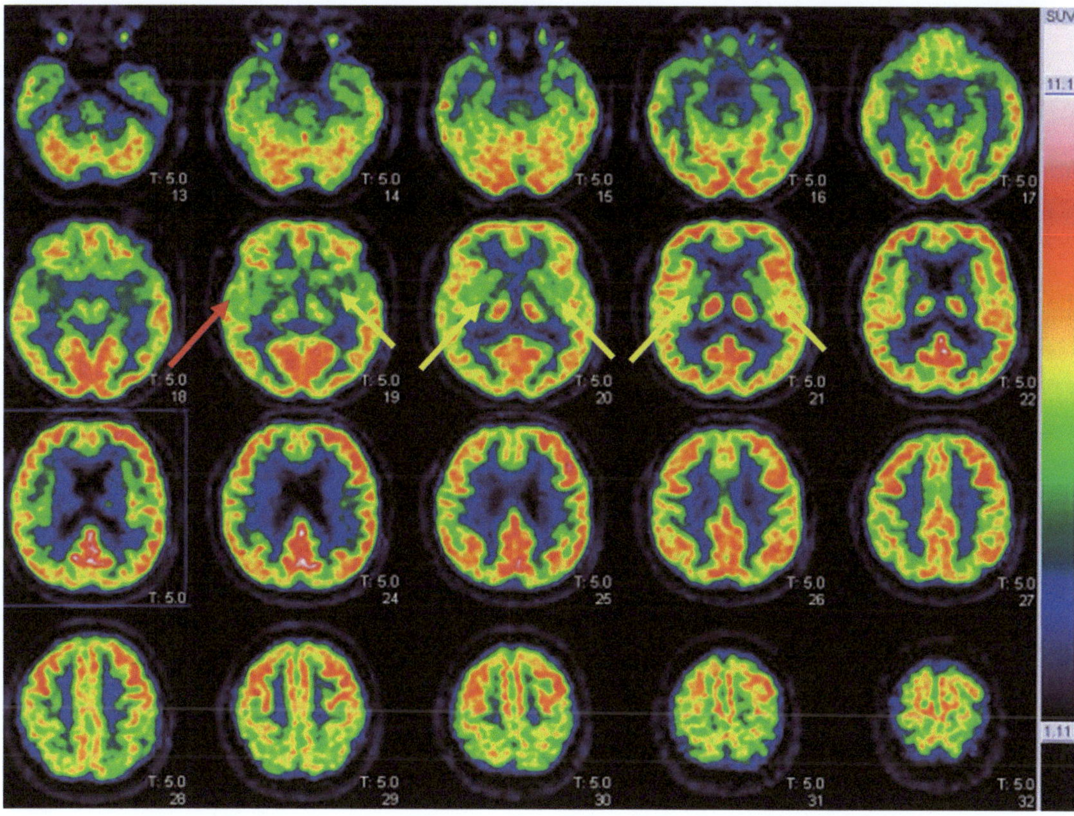


**Fig. 2** Axial brain FDG-PET images

## Imaging Findings

- Symptomatic HD patients show bilateral hypometabolism involving the striatum. Striatal hypometabolism may be an earlier finding as compared to striatal volume loss on MRI.
- Bilateral increase in thalamic, occipital, and cerebellar FDG uptake has also been identified as a typical feature of HD.
- Frontal-lobe hypometabolism responsible for cognitive deterioration has also been described in symptomatic HD patients.
- The same FDG uptake pattern has been described in premanifest HD gene carriers.

**Take Home Messages**

- A careful investigation of motor abnormalities is needed in psychiatric patients.
- Severely reduced glucose metabolism in the bilateral striatum is a well-described (and characteristic) neuroimaging finding in HD.
- In cases with negative family history the HD characteristic metabolic pattern can lead to the diagnosis when no other dementia-suspected (cortical) changes are present.

## Further Reading


Agosta F, Altomare D, Festari C, Orini S, Gandolfo F, Boccardi M, et al. EANM-EAN Task force for the prescription of FDG-PET for dementing neurodegenerative disorders. Clinical utility of FDG-PET in amyotrophic lateral sclerosis and Huntington's disease. Eur J Nucl Med Mol Imaging. 2018;45:1546–56.

Antonini A, Leenders KL, Spiegel R, Meier D, Vontobel P, WeigellWeber M, et al. Striatal glucose metabolism and dopamine D2 receptor binding in asymptomatic gene carriers and patients with Huntington's disease. Brain. 1996;119:2085–95.

Ciarmiello A, Cannella M, Lastoria S, Simonelli M, Frati L, Rubinsztein DC, et al. Brain white-matter volume loss and glucose hypometabolism precede the clinical symptoms of Huntington's disease. J Nucl Med. 2006;47:215–22.

Feigin A, Tang C, Ma Y, Mattis P, Zgaljardic D, Guttman M, et al. Thalamic metabolism and symptom onset in preclinical Huntington's disease. Brain. 2007;130:2858–67.

Kuwert T, Lange HW, Langen KJ, Herzog H, Aulich A, Feinendegen LE. Cortical and subcortical glucose consumption measured by PET in patients with Huntington's disease. Brain. 1990;113:1405–23.

Young AB, Penney JB, Starosta-Rubinstein S, Markel DS, Berent S, Giordani B, et al. PET scan investigations of Huntington's disease: cerebral metabolic correlates of neurological features and functional decline. Ann Neurol. 1986;20(3):296–303.

# Case 14: Creutzfeldt–Jakob Disease with Pathological Confirmation

Javier Arbizu and Juan Jose Rosales

## Case Summary

A 71-year-old male with no relevant medical history was admitted at the emergency room referring instability, dizziness, anxiety and insomnia over the last month and a half. His general practitioner physician, who initially evaluated him, prescribed Sulpiride and Lorazepam. Unfortunately, he became more anxious with distal tremor and got worse, so he stopped the medication with clinical improvement of some symptoms. Since 2 weeks ago, his relatives also referred behavioral changes and inability to perform basic activities of daily life. Additionally, he revealed loss of memory and a feeling of strangeness on the right hand and visual disturbances.

On physical examination, patient was awake and collaborative. His conversation was often disrupted by spontaneous confabulations. Cranial nerve evaluation was normal and no cerebellar signs were seen.

General blood tests were normal. The brain CT performed ruled out an acute vascular bleeding or ischemic lesions, and brain tumor neoplasm. Nevertheless, the patient showed a marked brain atrophy (more than expected by his age). Finally, he was admitted in our hospital for further evaluation.

## Images/Findings

The initial brain MRI scan displayed a diffuse brain atrophy and marked lateral ventricles enlargement that suggested subcortical atrophy or normal pressure hydrocephalus. The isolated white matter hyperintensities observed on the $T_2$-weighted fluid-attenuated inversion recovery (FLAIR) sequences were considered adjusted to the patient age (Fig. 1). Unfortunately, the patient did not collaborate during the scan acquisition and an additional brain MRI should be performed the day after. In this second scan, there were mild sings of restricted diffusion (hyperintensity) on the diffusion-weighted sequences (DWI) in the calcarine, cuneus, cingulate and parieto-occipital cortices (Fig. 2).

On the same day, a brain [$^{18}$F]fluorodeoxyglucose Positron Emission Tomography study (FDG-PET) was performed for further evaluation (Fig. 3). An extensive posterior cortical hypometabolism in the left hemisphere affecting parietal, occipital, calcarine, posterior cingulate and lateral temporal lobes. Interestingly, the hypometabolism area extended beyond the area of

J. Arbizu (✉) · J. J. Rosales
Department of Nuclear Medicine, Clinica Universidad de Navarra, University of Navarra, Pamplona, Spain
e-mail: jarbizu@unav.es


A. Varrone et al. (eds.), *Clinical Nuclear Medicine in Neurology*,
https://doi.org/10.1007/978-3-030-83598-9_14

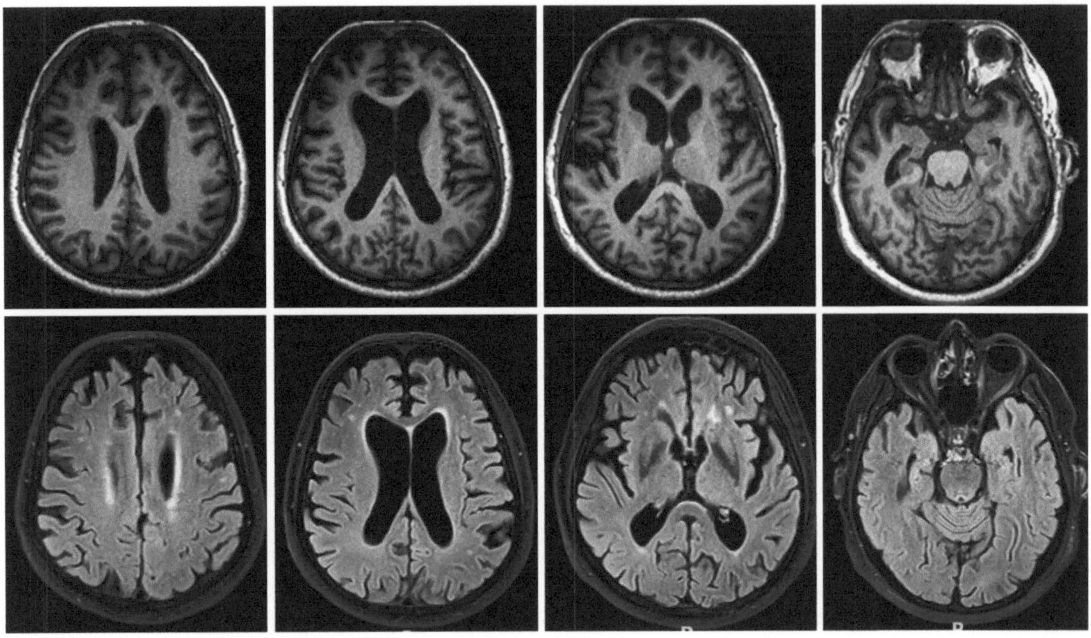

**Fig. 1** Axial slices of brain MRI scan. The $T_1$-weighted sequence (upper row) shows a diffuse brain atrophy and the enlargement of lateral ventricles, without any tumoral neoplasia or vascular infarcts. The $T_2$-FLAIR sequence (lower row) only displays occasional white matter hyperintensities of presumed vascular origin (leukoaraiosis), without any cortical hyperintensities suggesting lesion or disturbance

hyperintensity observed in the DWI sequences of the MRI. In addition, there was a moderate hypometabolism in the dorsolateral and medial frontal cortex that appeared normal on the DWI and FLAIR-MRI sequences. Important to note was the subcortical hypometabolism in the left thalamus and left caudate (Fig. 3).

EEG showed slow delta waves on left hemisphere predominantly on the frontotemporal area, which occasionally adopted a triphasic morphology.

The analysis of cerebral spinal fluid (CSF) obtained after lumbar puncture did not disclose an increase of cellularity (1 cell/μL), while the glucose (70 mg/dL) and proteins (29.73 mg/dL) levels were within the normal values. The presence of 14-3-3 protein in CSF was negative (method of Hsich). On the other hand, and extended serology analysis was negative.

Patient progressed to a clear deterioration state with disorganized and chaotic behavior, and lack of cognitive competence, fulfilling the syndromic diagnosis of rapidly progressive dementia and etiological diagnosis of probable sporadic Creutzfeldt–Jakob disease (sCJD). The patient received supportive care treatment with unfavorable clinical evolution dying less than 2 months after the first consultation. Post-mortem brain necropsy revealed spongiform changes and astrocytic gliosis consistent with the neuropathological diagnosis of sCJD.

## Diagnosis

Rapidly progressive dementia due to sCJD.

## Discussion

sCJD represents approximately 85% among all prion diseases [1]. This entity is believed to be caused by an abnormal isoform of a cellular glycoprotein known as the prion protein. A rapidly progressive dementia, ataxia and myoclonic involuntary movements characterize the clinical syndrome. The mean age at onset is 64 years and the mean duration is 6 months with less than 10% of subjects living more than 1 year.

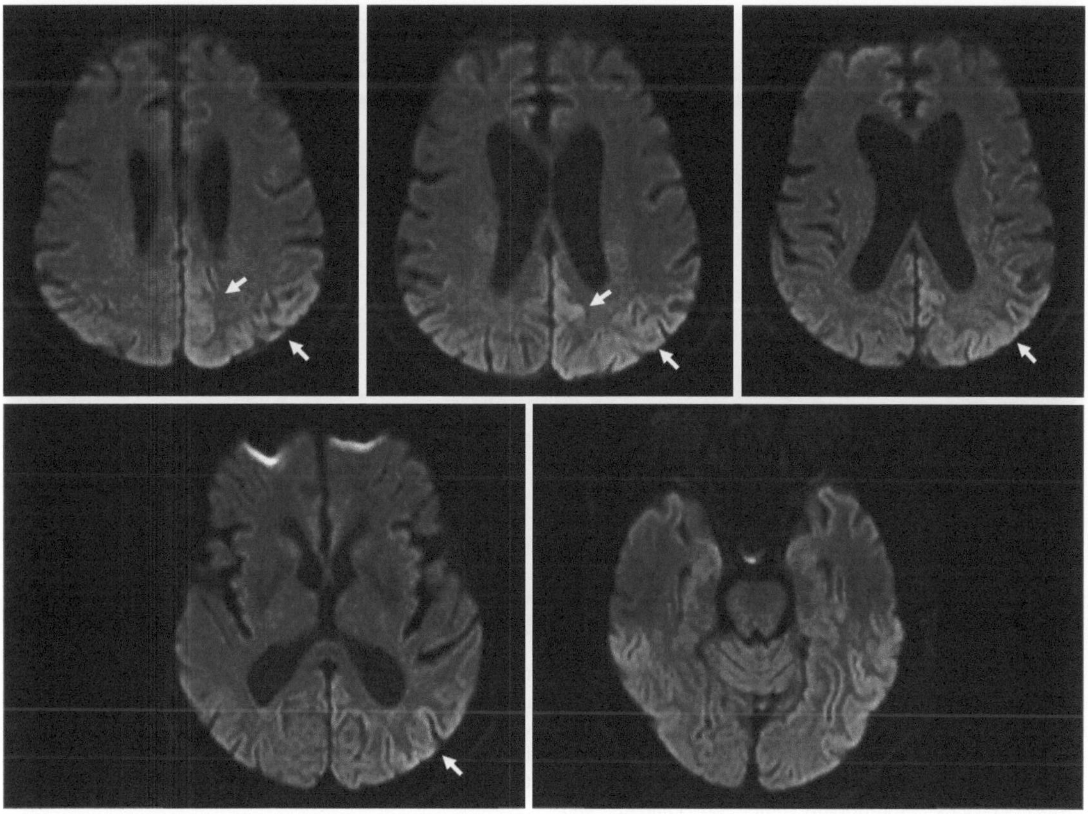

**Fig. 2** Axial slices of DWI brain MRI sequence. There is a mild restricted diffusion (hyperintensity) on the left posterior parietal, calcarine and posterior cingulate (white arrows in the upper row), and lateral temporo-occipital cortex (white arrow on the lower row). The remainder cortical and subcortical encephalic structures display a normal signal

Diagnosis can be challenging since symptoms are variable and common to other neurological conditions. Definitive diagnosis can only be made by pathological confirmation. Probability criteria are based on the presence of clinical features and complementary test such us electroencephalogram, detection of 14-3-3 protein in CSF and MRI findings according to the 2018 Guidelines published by Centers for Disease Control and Prevention [2]. MRI findings in sCJD include high signal changes in the cerebral cortex, basal ganglia or thalamus on FLAIR and DWIs sequences, and they have high sensitivity and specificity for sCJD, even in the early stage of the disease [3]. A positive immunoassay for the 14-3-3 brain protein in cerebrospinal fluid strongly supports a diagnosis of CJD in patients with clinically evident dementia [4]. However, a negative result makes the diagnosis of CJD unlikely, but does not rule out it. The EEG usually shows a typical repetitive pattern of bilateral synchronous periodic epileptiform discharges such as triphasic waves.

In our case, the standard complementary test were not particularly helpful as MRI showed mild hyperintensities only in DWI sequence, and the EEG and the 14-3-3 brain protein in CSF were negative. However, the pattern of hypometabolism in the FDG-PET was highly suggestive of sCJD and helped a further evaluation of the MRI images. Although FDG-PET imaging is not included in the diagnosis criteria yet, it might have a significant role in the diagnosis of prion diseases [5]. Patients with CJD

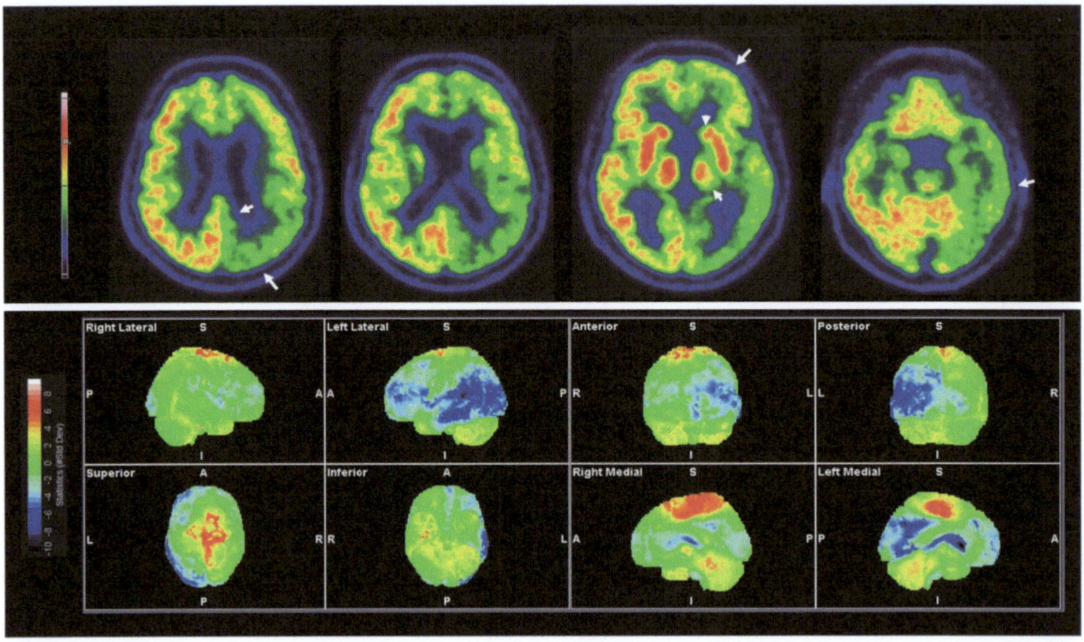


**Fig. 3** [[18]F]FDG-PET scan. In the axial slices (upper row), there is an extensive and marked hypometabolism (white arrows) that involves parietal, calcarine, posterior cingulate lateral temporal, with a moderate hypometabolism of the dorsolateral frontal cortex including operculo-insular cortices. Additionally, the left caudate and thalamus look hypometabolic (white arrows). The statistical surface projections after normal database comparison display areas of significant hypometabolism (>2 SD in blue) and hypermetabolism (>2 SD in red) in the primary and supplementary motor cortices

show a pattern of symmetrical hypometabolism in subcortical structures (thalamus, basal ganglia or both), as well as an asymmetric patched cortical hypometabolism [5, 6]. In some cases, an asymmetric distribution of FDG in basal ganglia can been seen in patients with sCJD presenting with corticobasal syndrome, which can be mistaken for a corticobasal degeneration (CBD) pattern [7]. Therefore, FDG-PET brain scan can be of particular interest in the early stages of rapidly progressive dementia syndrome when sCJD is suspected and the MRI scan is normal or unclear. Moreover, the clinical circumstances of sCJD patients make collaboration during the MRI scan acquisition difficult and, consequently, they can limitate the interpretation of DWI sequences.

Unfortunately, no specific therapy is currently available to stop the progression of prion diseases, and treatment remains supportive [8].

## Conclusions

FDG-PET imaging might play and important role in the early diagnosis of sCJD, as changes in the metabolic activity of cortical and subcortical structures may precede anatomical changes seen on MRI, an thus help to support clinical suspicion specially when the diagnosis remains unclear.

## References

1. Fragoso DC, Gonçalves Filho AL, Pacheco FT, Barros BR, Aguiar Littig I, Nunes RH, et al. Imaging of Creutzfeldt-Jakob disease: imaging patterns and their differential diagnosis. Radiographics. 2017;37:234–57.
2. CDC. Diagnostic criteria. Creutzfeldt-Jakob Disease. Classic (CJD). Prion disease. Atlanta, GA: CDC; 2018. https://www.cdc.gov/prions/cjd/diagnostic-criteria.html
3. Vitali P, Maccagnano E, Caverzasi E, Henry RG, Haman A, Torres-Chae C, et al. Diffusion-weighted

MRI hyperintensity patterns differentiate CJD from other rapid dementias. Neurology. 2011;76:1711–9.
4. Hsich G, Kenney K, Gibbs CJ, Lee KH, Harrington MG. The 14-3-3 brain protein in cerebrospinal fluid as a marker for transmissible spongiform encephalopathies. N Engl J Med. 1996;335(13):924–30.
5. Arbizu J, Giuliani A, Gállego Perez-Larraya J, Riverol M, Jonsson C, et al. Emerging clinical issues and multivariate analyses in PET investigations. Q J Nucl Med Mol Imaging. 2017;61:386–404.
6. Prieto E, Domínguez-Prado I, Riverol M, Ortega-Cubero S, Ribelles MJ, Luquin MR, et al. Metabolic patterns in prion diseases: an FDG PET voxel-based analysis. Eur J Nucl Med Mol Imaging. 2015;42(10):1522–9.
7. Zhang Y, Minoshima S, Vesselle H, Lewis DH. A case of Creutzfeldt-Jakob disease mimicking corticobasal degeneration. Clin Nucl Med. 2012;37:e173–5.
8. Paterson RW, Takada LT, Geschwind MD. Diagnosis and treatment of rapidly progressive dementias. Neurol Clin Pract. 2012;2:187–200.

# Section II

# Nuclear Medicine Cases of Epilepsy and Encephalitis

# Case 15: Non-lesional Temporal Epilepsy

Valentina Garibotto, Maria Isabel Vargas, John O. Prior, Andrea O. Rossetti, Serge Vulliemoz, and Margitta Seeck

## Introduction

2-[$^{18}$F]fluoro-2-deoxy-D-glucose ([$^{18}$F]FDG) PET imaging is an important tool for the presurgical assessment of patients with drug-resistant epilepsy and has shown an added value in cases without lesions visible on Magnetic resonance Imaging (MRI), defined as non-lesional epilepsy [1]. Importantly, non-lesional [$^{18}$F]FDG-positive cases might have a favorable prognosis and surgical outcome, comparable to lesional cases [2–4].

The detection of abnormalities on [$^{18}$F]FDG PET images relies on a combination of visual analysis and automated analysis tools. The visual assessment has a high sensitivity, but remains subjective and depends on the level of expertise of the reader. The automated tools are usually based on the statistical comparison with a reference database, and have been shown to usefully support visual interpretation, namely in cases of extra-temporal epilepsy [5]. Both for visual and semi-quantitative assessment, detecting a left/right asymmetry may contribute to the localization of the epileptogenic focus [6, 7].

V. Garibotto (✉)
Division of Nuclear Medicine and Molecular Imaging, Diagnostic Department, University Hospitals of Geneva, Geneva, Switzerland

Faculty of Medicine, University of Geneva, Geneva, Switzerland
e-mail: Valentina.Garibotto@hcuge.ch

M. I. Vargas
Faculty of Medicine, University of Geneva, Geneva, Switzerland

Division of Neuroradiology, Diagnostic Department, University Hospitals of Geneva, Geneva, Switzerland
e-mail: maria.i.vargas@hcuge.ch

J. O. Prior
Department of Nuclear Medicine and Molecular Imaging, Lausanne University Hospital (CHUV), University of Lausanne, Lausanne, Switzerland
e-mail: john.prior@chuv.ch

A. O. Rossetti
Department of Clinical Neuroscience, Lausanne University Hospital (CHUV), University of Lausanne, Lausanne, Switzerland
e-mail: andrea.rossetti@chuv.ch

S. Vulliemoz · M. Seeck
Faculty of Medicine, University of Geneva, Geneva, Switzerland

Neurology Department, University Hospitals of Geneva, Geneva, Switzerland
e-mail: serge.vulliemoz@hcuge.ch; margitta.seeck@hcuge.ch


A. Varrone et al. (eds.), *Clinical Nuclear Medicine in Neurology*,
https://doi.org/10.1007/978-3-030-83598-9_15

## Case Presentation

A 38-year-old woman with a 5 years history of pharmaco-resistant focal seizures with autonomic symptoms with secondary bilateralization was evaluated for a curative surgery.

The interictal electroencephalography (EEG) showed a right temporal abnormality, accentuated during sleep. The ictal EEG recording showed bilateral anterior temporal abnormalities, predominant on the right side. The neuropsychological evaluation identified a more pronounced visual than verbal memory impairment.

## Methods

MRI imaging was performed on a 3 T scanner with a standardized clinical protocol.

[$^{18}$F]FDG PET imaging was performed 30 min after injection of 194 MBq of [$^{18}$F]FDG, during the interictal phase, following current procedural guidelines [8].

## Imaging Findings

MRI was normal, both at visual and volumetric assessment, without any right temporal abnormality.

[$^{18}$F]FDG PET images showed a slight anterior temporal asymmetry at visual evaluation (Fig. 1).

A standardized comparison with a normal reference database showed that the metabolism of the anterior temporal region was within normal ranges, with only a slight asymmetry as compared to the contralateral hemisphere (the asymmetry index was 7%, still within normal values, i.e., below 15%) (Fig. 2).

## Follow-Up Information

The patient underwent a right amygdalo-hippocampectomy. The pathological analysis of the resected tissue identified changes consistent with a focal cortical dysplasia. At 2 years follow-up, a marked improvement in her seizures' frequency was observed (Engel Class III).

**Take Home Message**

[$^{18}$F]FDG PET has an added value in non-lesional epilepsy cases. Metabolic abnormalities might be subtle and the combination of visual and automated analyses, namely assessing carefully the presence of any asymmetry and taking into account EEG and seizure semiology, can greatly contribute to image interpretation.

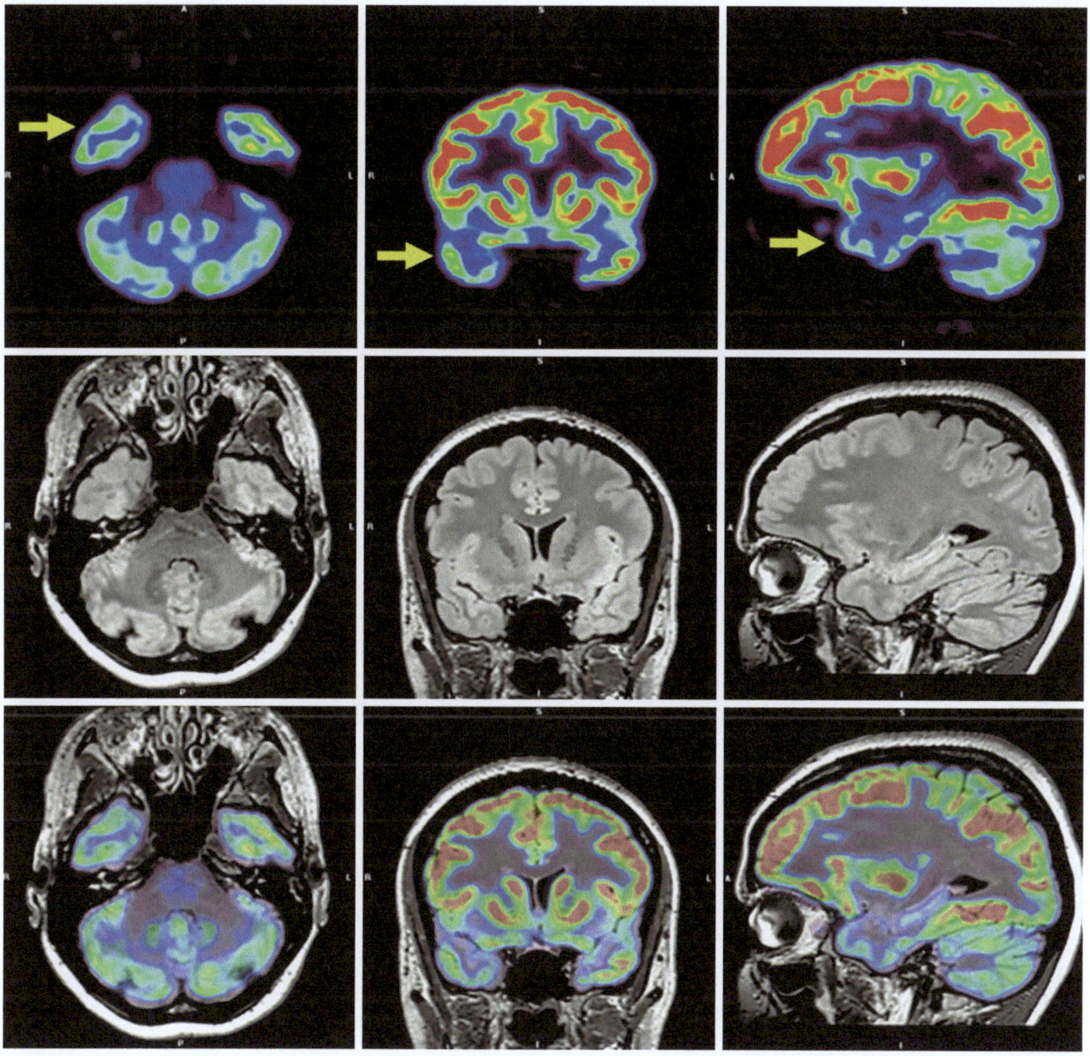

**Fig. 1** The visual analysis of the [$^{18}$F]FDG PET distribution shows an asymmetric metabolism in the anterior temporo-polar region, as indicated by the yellow arrow (upper row: PET images; middle row: 3D FLAIR MRI images; lower row: PET-MRI fusion)

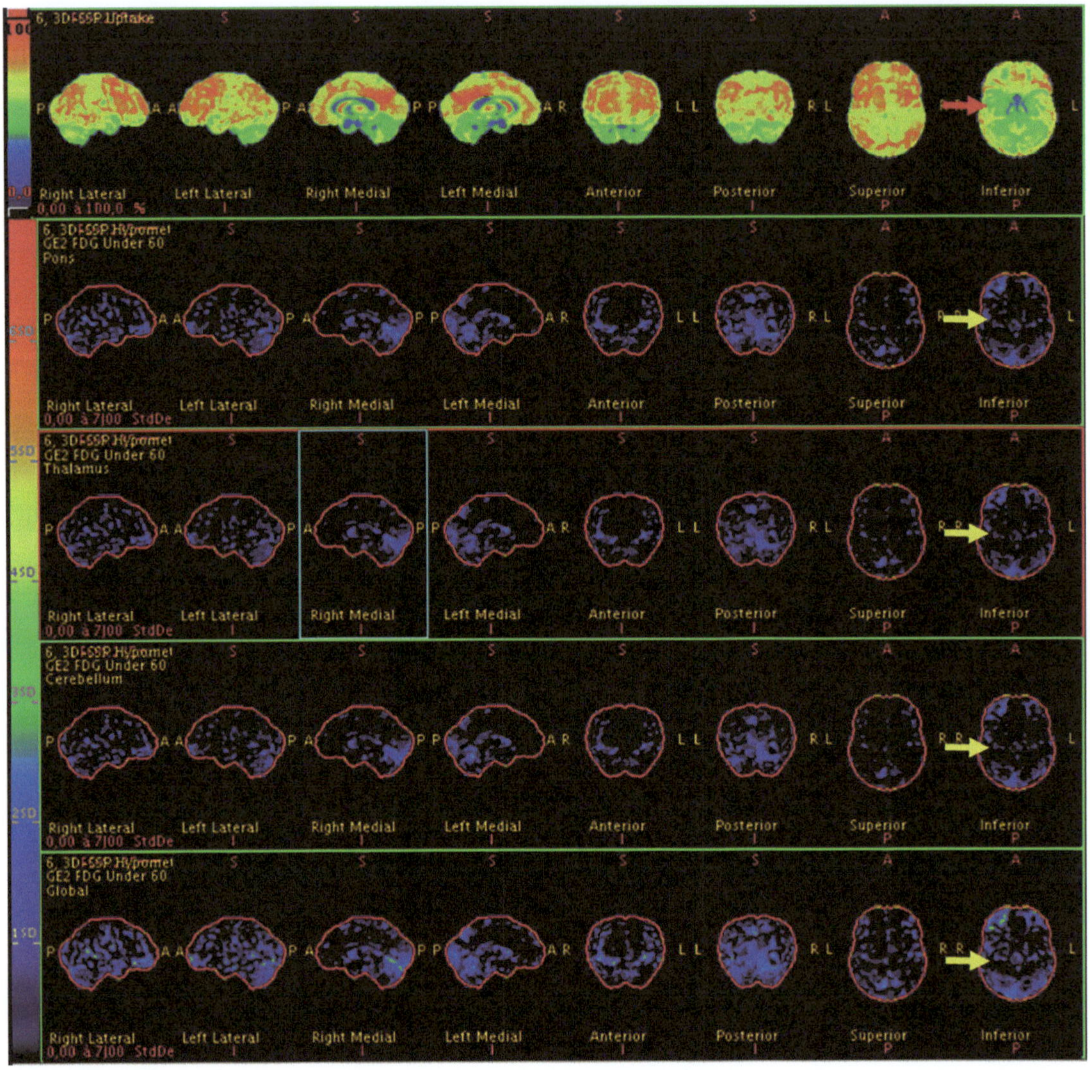


**Fig. 2** The slight reduction in tracer uptake visible in the right anterior temporal region (red arrow) did not correspond to any significant change at the standardized comparison with a normal reference database (Cortex ID software, yellow arrows indicating the lack of significant findings in this region independently on the region used for normalization)

## References


1. Carne RP, O'Brien TJ, Kilpatrick CJ, MacGregor LR, Hicks RJ, Murphy MA, Bowden SC, Kaye AH, Cook MJ. MRI-negative PET-positive temporal lobe epilepsy: a distinct surgically remediable syndrome. Brain. 2004;127(Pt 10):2276–85.
2. Tomas J, Pittau F, Hammers A, Bouvard S, Picard F, Vargas MI, Sales F, Seeck M, Garibotto V. The predictive value of hypometabolism in focal epilepsy: a prospective study in surgical candidates. Eur J Nucl Med Mol Imaging. 2019;46(9):1806–16.
3. Thorsteinsdottir J, Vollmar C, Tonn JC, Kreth FW, Noachtar S, Peraud A. Outcome after individualized stereoelectroencephalography (sEEG) implantation and navigated resection in patients with lesional and non-lesional focal epilepsy. J Neurol. 2019;266(4):910–20.
4. Kogias E, Klingler JH, Urbach H, Scheiwe C, Schmeiser B, Doostkam S, Zentner J, Altenmuller DM. 3 Tesla MRI-negative focal epilepsies: presurgi-

cal evaluation, postoperative outcome and predictive factors. Clin Neurol Neurosurg. 2017;163:116–20.
5. Mendes Coelho VC, Morita ME, Amorim BJ, Ramos CD, Yasuda CL, Tedeschi H, Ghizoni E, Cendes F. Automated online quantification method for (18) F-FDG positron emission tomography/CT improves detection of the epileptogenic zone in patients with pharmacoresistant epilepsy. Front Neurol. 2017;8:453.
6. Lin TW, de Aburto MA, Dahlbom M, Huang LL, Marvi MM, Tang M, Czernin J, Phelps ME, Silverman DH. Predicting seizure-free status for temporal lobe epilepsy patients undergoing surgery: prognostic value of quantifying maximal metabolic asymmetry extending over a specified proportion of the temporal lobe. J Nucl Med. 2007;48(5):776–82.
7. Soma T, Momose T, Takahashi M, Koyama K, Kawai K, Murase K, Ohtomo K. Usefulness of extent analysis for statistical parametric mapping with asymmetry index using inter-ictal FGD-PET in mesial temporal lobe epilepsy. Ann Nucl Med. 2012;26(4):319–26.
8. Varrone A, Asenbaum S, Vander Borght T, Booij J, Nobili F, Nagren K, Darcourt J, Kapucu OL, Tatsch K, Bartenstein P, et al. EANM procedure guidelines for PET brain imaging using [18F]FDG, version 2. Eur J Nucl Med Mol Imaging. 2009;36(12):2103–10.

# Case 16: Ictal [18F]FDG PET Imaging

Valentina Garibotto, Christian Korff, Maria Isabel Vargas, Serge Vulliemoz, and Margitta Seeck

## Introduction

2-[$^{18}$F]fluoro-2-deoxy-D-glucose ([$^{18}$F]FDG) PET imaging is an established imaging modality in the pre-surgical evaluation of epilepsy [1]. [$^{18}$F]FDG PET is usually performed during the interictal condition, while SPECT perfusion is preferred for imaging in ictal phase for a number of considerations, namely faster tracer uptake, lower redistribution and longer half-life.

However, [$^{18}$F]FDG PET imaging in ictal phase, although rarely obtained, can be obtained namely in patients with continuous or very frequent focal seizures [2]. In these cases the superior spatial resolution of the technology, as compared with SPECT, can provide a high quality picture of the seizure onset zone and of its network.

[$^{18}$F]FDG PET imaging in patients with Rasmussen encephalitis has been previously reported, usually showing a hemispheric hypometabolism associated with atrophy and, less frequently, focal hypermetabolism linked to seizure activity [3].

## Case Presentation

Drug-resistant focal epilepsy in a 5-year-old patient with Rasmussen encephalitis diagnosed 2 years earlier and s left hemispheric focal seizures.

The evaluation is motivated by a sudden increase in seizure frequency, now almost continuous (as shown in Fig. 1), and worsening of language performance despite adequate phar-

V. Garibotto (✉)
Division of Nuclear Medicine and Molecular Imaging, Diagnostic Department, University Hospitals of Geneva, Geneva, Switzerland

Faculty of Medicine, University of Geneva, Geneva, Switzerland
e-mail: Valentina.Garibotto@hcuge.ch

C. Korff
Faculty of Medicine, University of Geneva, Geneva, Switzerland

Pediatric Neurology Unit, Department of the Woman, Child and Adolescent, University Hospitals of Geneva, Geneva, Switzerland
e-mail: Christian.Korff@hcuge.ch

M. I. Vargas
Faculty of Medicine, University of Geneva, Geneva, Switzerland

Division of Neuroradiology, Diagnostic Department, University Hospitals of Geneva, Geneva, Switzerland
e-mail: maria.i.vargas@hcuge.ch

S. Vulliemoz · M. Seeck
Faculty of Medicine, University of Geneva, Geneva, Switzerland

Neurology Department, University Hospitals of Geneva, Geneva, Switzerland
e-mail: serge.vulliemoz@hcuge.ch; margitta.seeck@hcuge.ch


A. Varrone et al. (eds.), *Clinical Nuclear Medicine in Neurology*,
https://doi.org/10.1007/978-3-030-83598-9_16

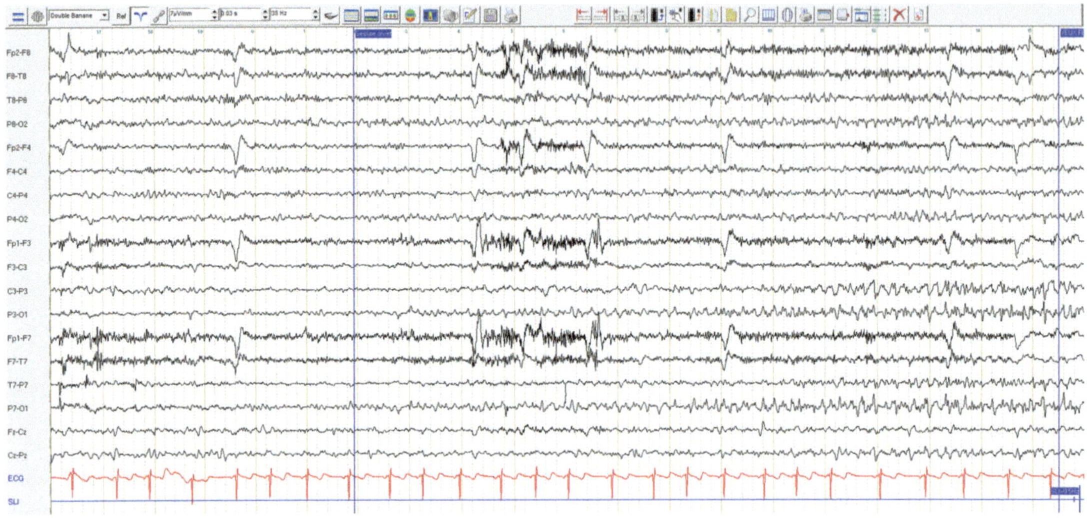


**Fig. 1** EEG: Seizure onset with recruiting rhythmic activity (spikes and beta activity) in the left parieto-occipital region (EEG onset marked)

macological treatment of four different medications.

A functional left hemispherotomy is planned and imaging is performed to confirm the integrity of the contralateral hemisphere.

## Methods

[$^{18}$F]FDG PET imaging was performed 30 min after injection of 117 MBq of [$^{18}$F]FDG, following current procedural guidelines [4].

The injection was performed with electroencephalographic (EEG) monitoring showing left parieto-occipital "epilepsia partialis continua."

## Imaging Findings

[$^{18}$F]FDG PET images (Figs. 2 and 3) showed:

- a diffuse left hemispheric hypometabolism, mostly visible at the insular and temporal level,
- a bifocal left hemisphere hypermetabolism of the premotor and parieto-occipital cortex,
- a focal hypermetabolism of the left thalamus,
- a bifocal hypermetabolism of the right cerebellar hemisphere, reflecting crossed cerebellar activation [5].

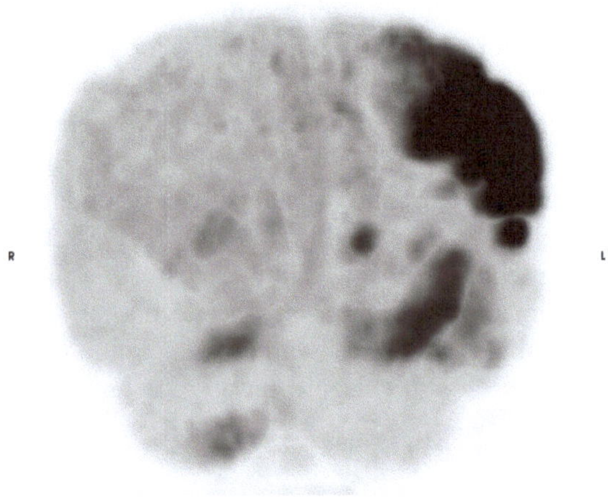


**Fig. 2** [$^{18}$F]FDG PET 3D maximum intensity projection (MIP) image showing that hyperactivity was limited to the left cerebral hemisphere and to the contralateral cerebellar hemisphere

## Follow-Up Information

The patient underwent left hemispherotomy. At biopsy the hippocampal tissue showed inflammatory changes consistent with Rasmussen encephalitis.

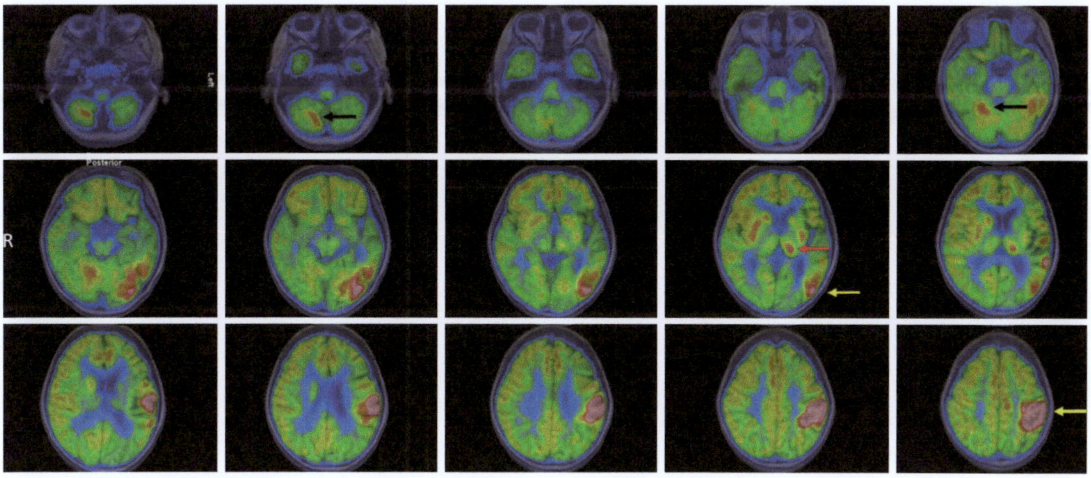


**Fig. 3** [$^{18}$F]FDG PET/MRI fusion images showing the anatomical localization of the two foci of hypermetabolism on the left hemisphere (yellow arrows), as well as the focal uptake of the left thalamus (red arrow) and of the right cerebellum (black arrows)

The patient was seizure free 6 months after surgery, with progressive withdrawal of all antiepileptic drugs and with an encouraging cognitive and language development.

**Take Home Messages**

- EEG recording at the time of [$^{18}$F]FDG injection and uptake is required to correctly interpret PET images.
- Ictal [$^{18}$F]FDG imaging performed during frequent/continuous seizures depicts the epileptic activity with high spatial resolution and helps to verify the preservation of the contralateral hemisphere, crucial for a successful hemispheric disconnecting surgery.

## References

1. Mouthaan BE, Rados M, Barsi P, Boon P, Carmichael DW, Carrette E, Craiu D, Cross JH, Diehl B, Dimova P, et al. Current use of imaging and electromagnetic source localization procedures in epilepsy surgery centers across Europe. Epilepsia. 2016;57(5):770–6.
2. Meltzer CC, Adelson PD, Brenner RP, Crumrine PK, Van Cott A, Schiff DP, Townsend DW, Scheuer ML. Planned ictal FDG PET imaging for localization of extratemporal epileptic foci. Epilepsia. 2000;41(2):193–200.
3. Fiorella DJ, Provenzale JM, Coleman RE, Crain BJ, Al-Sugair AA. (18)F-fluorodeoxyglucose positron emission tomography and MR imaging findings in Rasmussen encephalitis. AJNR Am J Neuroradiol. 2001;22(7):1291–9.
4. Varrone A, Asenbaum S, Vander Borght T, Booij J, Nobili F, Nagren K, Darcourt J, Kapucu OL, Tatsch K, Bartenstein P, et al. EANM procedure guidelines for PET brain imaging using [18F]FDG, version 2. Eur J Nucl Med Mol Imaging. 2009;36(12):2103–10.
5. Kawai N, Kawanishi M, Tamiya T, Nagao S. Crossed cerebellar glucose hypermetabolism demonstrated using PET in symptomatic epilepsy—case report. Ann Nucl Med. 2005;19(3):231–4.

# Case 17: Focal Refractory Epilepsy with Negative MRI

Stanislas Lagarde, Tatiana Horowitz, and Eric Guedj

## Case Summary

A 20-year-old man was referred for drug-resistant epilepsy. He was a full-term infant, with no history of perinatal ischemia. Sleep-bound seizures were first noted at the age of 2. Seizures were stereotypic, characterized by dystonic arms movements, growling, and hindlimb clonus, uncontrolled after adequate trials of several anti-seizure medications. He was addressed for a pre-surgical evaluation. MRI did not reveal any epileptogenic lesion. Brain [$^{18}$F]FDG PET-CT among allowed to identify a focal metabolic defect, evocative of focal cortical dysplasia, with a focal epileptic zone confirmed by SEEG. The patient recovered after a tailored cortectomy and histology confirmed a focal cortical dysplasia.

A 20-year-old man with drug-resistant focal epilepsy and sleep-related hypermotor seizures (Figs. 1, 2 and 3).

The patient was operated (tailored cortectomy) within basal orbitofrontal area based on SEEG recordings. He is seizure-free for 4 years. Histology confirmed a focal cortical dysplasia.

## Epidemiology

- Focal epilepsies represent about 60% of all epilepsies.
- Among them about 30% are resistant to anti-seizure medication.
- In selected candidate (about 25%) epilepsy surgery can lead to about 50–75% of seizure-freedom.

## Pathology and Etiology

- Focal cortical dysplasia (FCD) are congenital malformations of cortical development.
- FCD are characterized by an histological disorganization of the cortical architecture more or less associated with abnormal (dysplastic) neurons.
- FCD are present in about 15% of the resection pieces in epilepsy surgery.
- FCD, especially type II, are good candidate for epilepsy surgery even in the case of normal MRI.

S. Lagarde · E. Guedj (✉)
Epileptology Department, Aix Marseille Univ, APHM, INSERM, INS, Inst Neurosci Syst, Timone Hospital, Marseille, France
e-mail: eric.guedj@univ-amu.fr

T. Horowitz
CERIMED, Nuclear Medicine Department, Aix Marseille Univ, APHM, CNRS, Centrale Marseille, Institut Fresnel, Timone Hospital, Marseille, France


A. Varrone et al. (eds.), *Clinical Nuclear Medicine in Neurology*,
https://doi.org/10.1007/978-3-030-83598-9_17

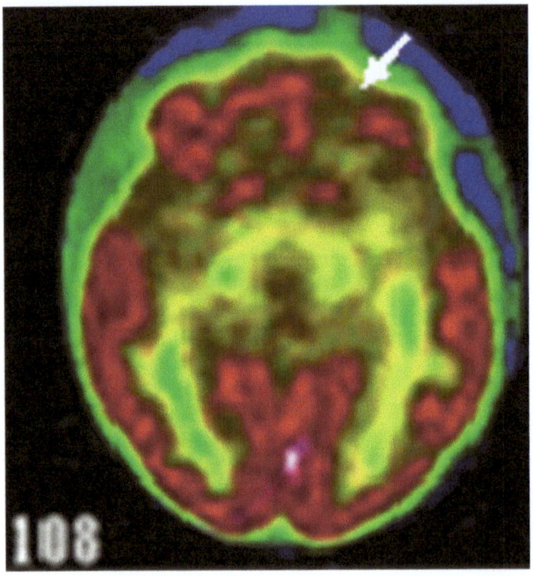


**Fig. 1** Axial PET images showing a focal right orbitofrontal [$^{18}$F]FDG decreased uptake, the rest of the cerebral glucose metabolism is normal

## Imaging Findings

- Nowadays the majority of patients (60–80%) addressed for potential epilepsy surgery has a negative MRI.
- Evocative FCD pattern on MRI shows cortical focal blurring (+/− transmantle sign, cortical thinning/thickening, …).
- [$^{18}$F]FDG PET can help to localize the epileptogenic zone showing area(s) of hypometabolism.
- MRI-PET fusion is particularly useful to localize the epileptogenic zone especially in case of focal cortical dysplasia.

**Take-Home Message**

- In MRI-negative focal drug-resistant epilepsy, [$^{18}$F]FDG PET-CT and particularly MRI-PET fusion can help, with the electroclinical investigation, to localize the epileptogenic zone.

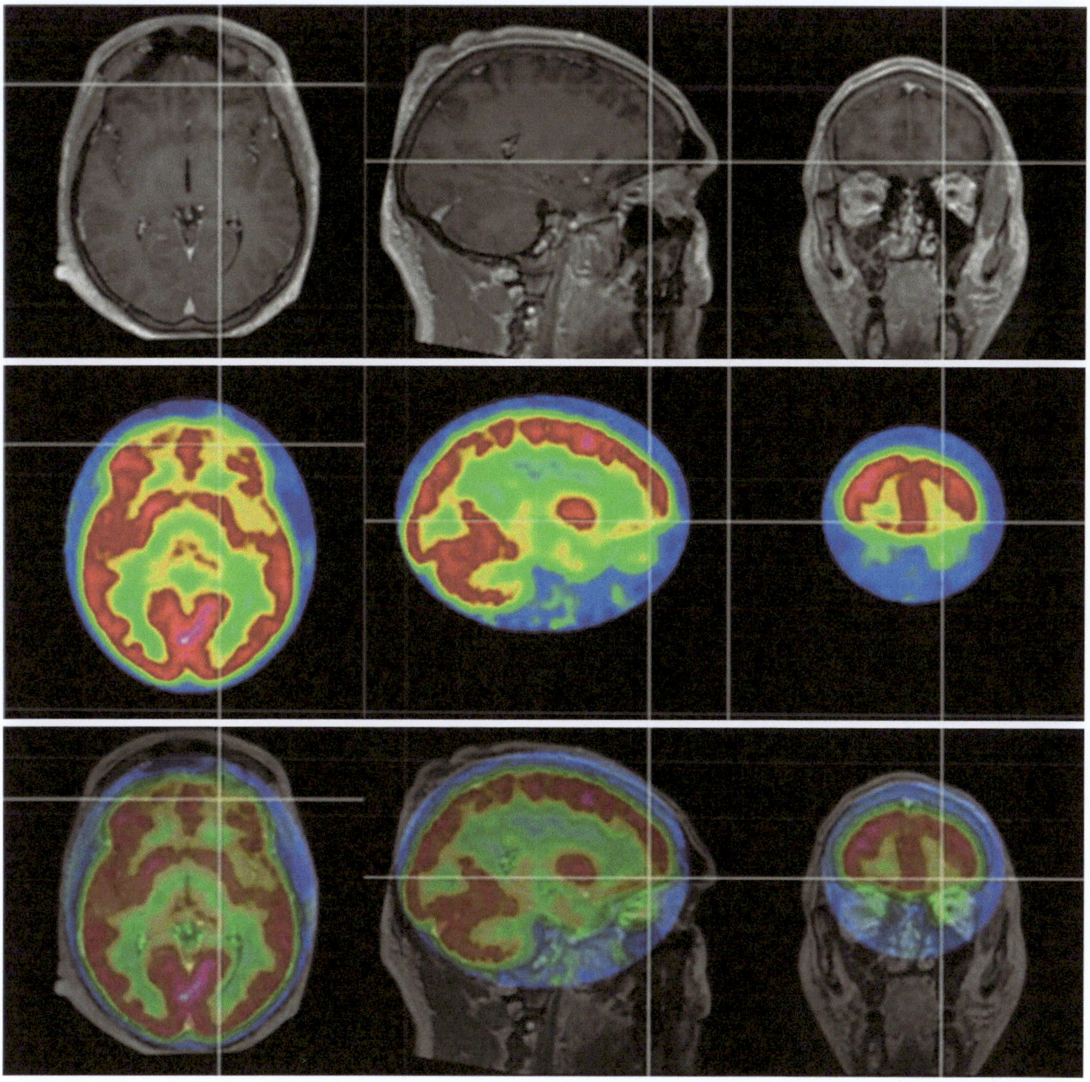

**Fig. 2** Corresponding [$^{18}$F]FDG PET-MRI fusion allows a more precise localization of the hypometabolic right fronto-orbital area

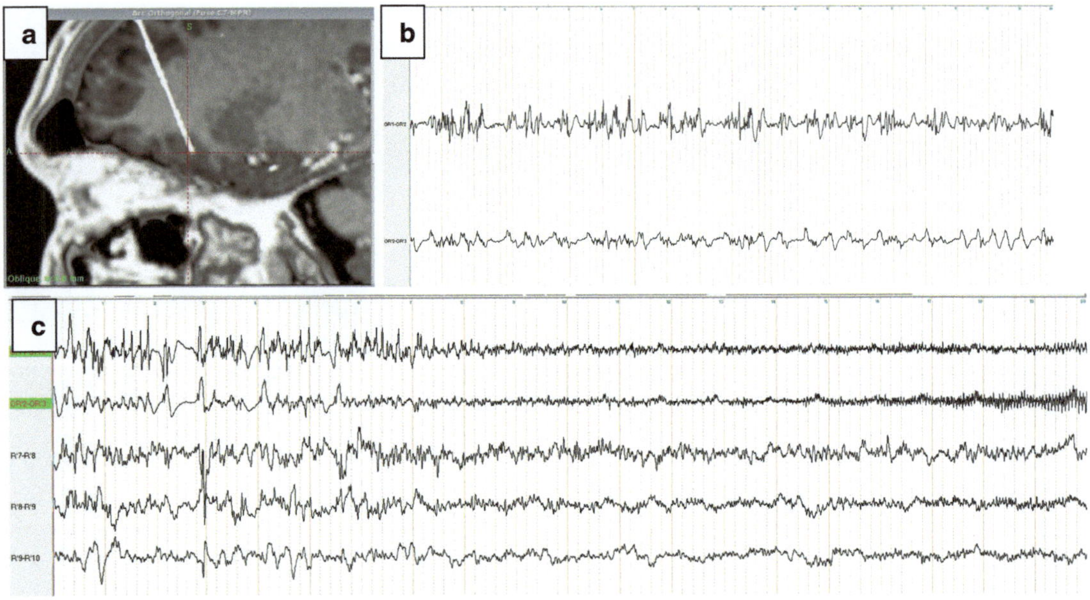


**Fig. 3** Intracerebral stereo-EEG recordings (SEEG) showing: (**a**) location of the electrode within the basal orbitofrontal region; (**b**) an interictal pattern of altered background activity with continuous periodic interictal epileptiform discharges evocative of focal cortical dysplasia within the basal orbitofrontal region; (**c**) ictal discharge with low voltage fast activity within the same area

## Further Reading

Chassoux F, Rodrigo S, Semah F, Beuvon F, Landre E, Devaux B, et al. FDG-PET improves surgical outcome in negative MRI Taylor-type focal cortical dysplasias. Neurology. 2010;75:2168–75.

Guerrini R, Duchowny M, Jayakar P, Krsek P, Kahane P, Tassi L, et al. Diagnostic methods and treatment options for focal cortical dysplasia. Epilepsia. 2015;56:1669–86.

Lagarde S, Boucekine M, McGonigal A, Carron R, Scavarda D, Trebuchon A, et al. Relationship between PET metabolism and SEEG epileptogenicity in focal lesional epilepsy. Eur J Nucl Med Mol Imaging. 2020;47(13):3130–42.

Verger A, Lagarde S, Maillard L, Bartolomei F, Guedj E. Brain molecular imaging in pharmacoresistant focal epilepsy: current practice and perspectives. Rev Neurol (Paris). 2018;174(1–2):16–27.

# Case 18: Metabolic Abnormalities After Failed Resective Temporal Epilepsy Surgery

Valentina Garibotto, Maria Isabel Vargas, Serge Vulliemoz, and Margitta Seeck

## Introduction

2-[$^{18}$F]fluoro-2-deoxy-D-glucose ([$^{18}$F]FDG) PET imaging is a well validated tool in patients with drug-resistant epilepsy and surgical candidates, considering its good diagnostic performance in the localization of the seizure onset zone, in combination with other imaging and electrophysiological methods [1]. The pattern of abnormalities identified on [$^{18}$F]FDG PET images reflects not only the epileptogenic lesion but also its associated network and might provide prognostic information [2].

The value of [$^{18}$F]FDG PET in cases with recurring seizures after a previous brain surgery is less established. In the literature, there are only a few case series reporting PET abnormalities in these cases, and there are no established criteria to evaluate which metabolic abnormalities in the periphery of the surgical cavity should be considered physiological or suspicious for residual epileptogenic tissue [3, 4].

## Case Presentation

We describe here a 20-year-old patient with a history of right temporal focal epilepsy and hippocampal sclerosis who had previously been treated by a selective right amygdala-hippocampectomy, now evaluated for seizures which recurred 5 years after surgery.

The clinical and electroencephalography (EEG) characteristics were comparable to the initial presentation and in favor of a mesial temporal origin.

V. Garibotto (✉)
Division of Nuclear Medicine and Molecular Imaging, Diagnostic Department, University Hospitals of Geneva, Geneva, Switzerland

Faculty of Medicine, University of Geneva, Geneva, Switzerland
e-mail: Valentina.Garibotto@hcuge.ch

M. I. Vargas
Faculty of Medicine, University of Geneva, Geneva, Switzerland

Division of Neuroradiology, Diagnostic Department, University Hospitals of Geneva, Geneva, Switzerland
e-mail: maria.i.vargas@hcuge.ch

S. Vulliemoz · M. Seeck
Faculty of Medicine, University of Geneva, Geneva, Switzerland

Neurology Department, University Hospitals of Geneva, Geneva, Switzerland
e-mail: serge.vulliemoz@hcuge.ch; margitta.seeck@hcuge.ch


A. Varrone et al. (eds.), *Clinical Nuclear Medicine in Neurology*,
https://doi.org/10.1007/978-3-030-83598-9_18

## Methods

Magnetic Resonance Imaging (MRI) was performed on a 3 Tesla scanner with a standardized clinical protocol [5].

[$^{18}$F]FDG PET imaging was performed 30 min after injection of 213 MBq of [$^{18}$F]FDG, during the interictal phase, as documented by EEG monitoring and following current procedural guidelines [6].

## Imaging Findings

MRI showed a residual portion of the right amygdala and of the posterior portion of the hippocampus (Figs. 1 and 2). The rest of the exam was normal.

[$^{18}$F]FDG PET images showed a severe hypometabolism of the residual hippocampus and amygdala, while the borders of the surgical cavity, namely in the lateral part of the temporal lobe, show physiological metabolism (Figs. 1 and 2).

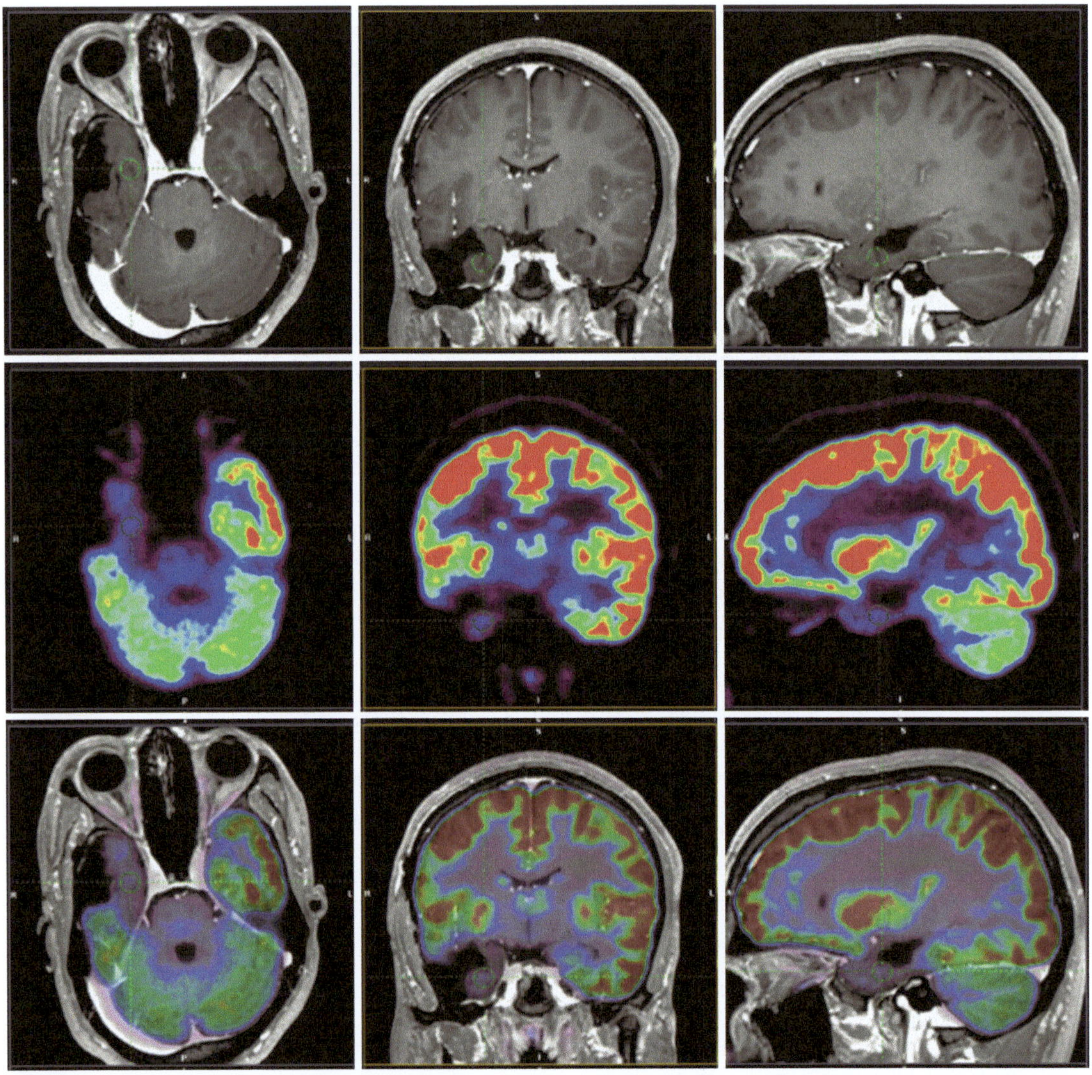

**Fig. 1** A residual portion of the temporomesial region was visible on the MRI images (upper row), as indicated by the crosshair. This region showed a severe hypometabolism (middle row: [$^{18}$F]FDG PET images, lower row: PET-MRI fusion)

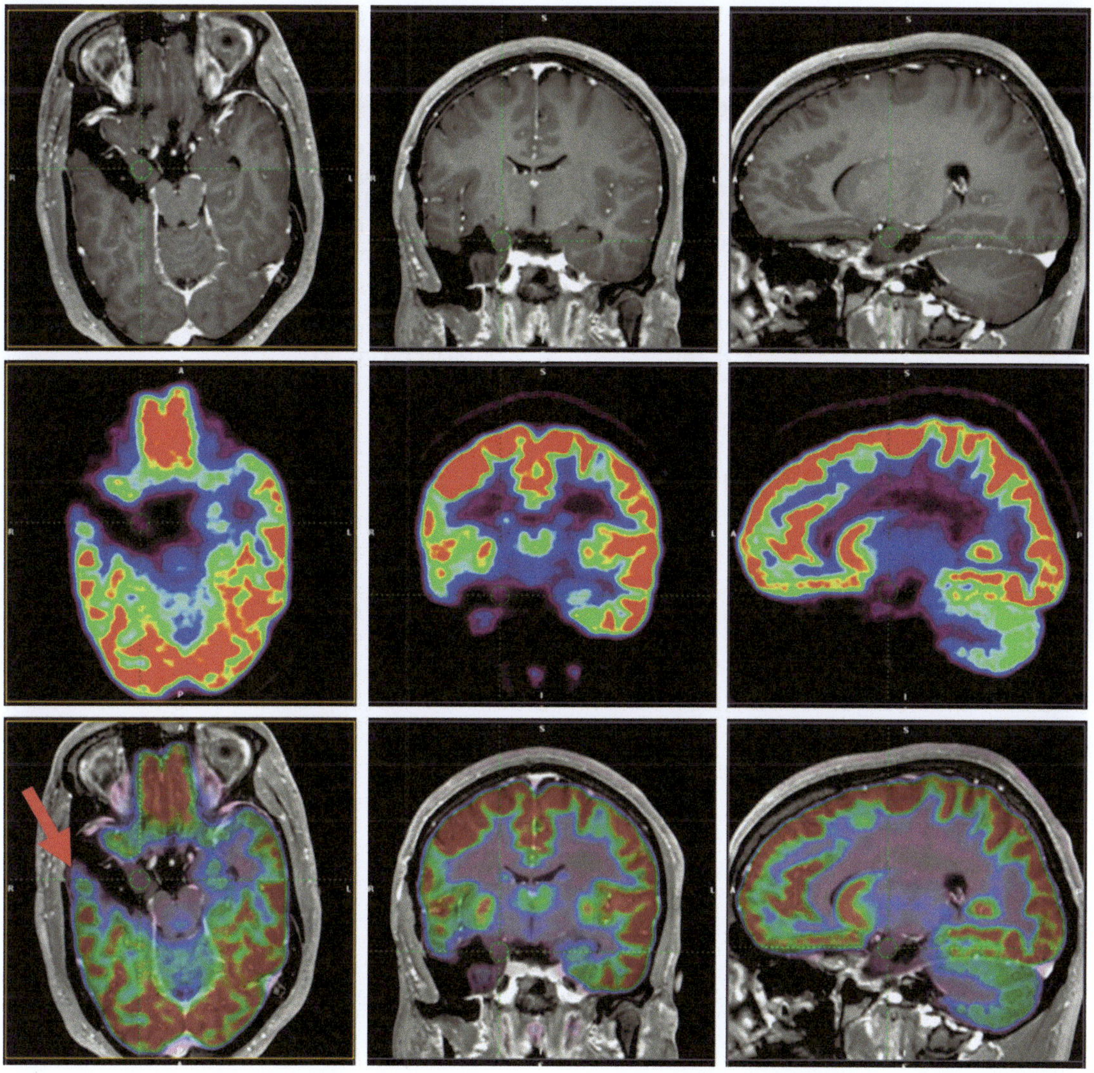

**Fig. 2** A residual portion of the right amygdala was visible on the MRI images (upper row), as indicated by the crosshair. This region showed a severe hypometabolism (middle row: [$^{18}$F]FDG PET images, lower row: PET-MRI fusion). The lateral temporal cortex shows instead a physiological metabolism (red arrow)

The severe hypometabolic pattern, together with a deficit in non-verbal memory was in favor of a severe dysfunction of these structures and suggested a low risk of cognitive deficit after their resection.

## Follow-Up Information

A second surgery was performed to remove the residual portions of amygdala and hippocampus: the patient was seizure-free at the first follow up evaluation with an improvement in non-verbal memory.

**Take Home Message**

- A focal hypometabolism of the structures surrounding the surgical cavity might contribute identifying the epileptogenic tissue. The combination of PET and MRI images, facilitated over the last years by the development of integrated systems, is of the utmost importance for the interpretation of PET findings in complex cases [7].

## References


1. Lascano AM, Perneger T, Vulliemoz S, Spinelli L, Garibotto V, Korff CM, Vargas MI, Michel CM, Seeck M. Yield of MRI, high-density electric source imaging (HD-ESI), SPECT and PET in epilepsy surgery candidates. Clin Neurophysiol. 2016;127(1):150–5.
2. Tomas J, Pittau F, Hammers A, Bouvard S, Picard F, Vargas MI, Sales F, Seeck M, Garibotto V. The predictive value of hypometabolism in focal epilepsy: a prospective study in surgical candidates. Eur J Nucl Med Mol Imaging. 2019;46(9):1806–16.
3. Surges R, Elger CE. Reoperation after failed resective epilepsy surgery. Seizure. 2013;22(7):493–501.
4. Reed CM, Dewar S, Fried I, Engel J Jr, Eliashiv D. Failed epilepsy surgery deserves a second chance. Clin Neurol Neurosurg. 2017;163:110–5.
5. Fitsiori A, Hiremath SB, Boto J, Garibotto V, Vargas MI. Morphological and advanced imaging of epilepsy: beyond the basics. Children (Basel). 2019;6(3):43.
6. Varrone A, Asenbaum S, Vander Borght T, Booij J, Nobili F, Nagren K, Darcourt J, Kapucu OL, Tatsch K, Bartenstein P, et al. EANM procedure guidelines for PET brain imaging using [18F]FDG, version 2. Eur J Nucl Med Mol Imaging. 2009;36(12):2103–10.
7. Grouiller F, Delattre BM, Pittau F, Heinzer S, Lazeyras F, Spinelli L, Iannotti GR, Seeck M, Ratib O, Vargas MI, et al. All-in-one interictal presurgical imaging in patients with epilepsy: single-session EEG/PET/(f)MRI. Eur J Nucl Med Mol Imaging. 2015;42(7):1133–43.

# Case 19: Hypothalamic Hamartoma with Cortical Metabolic Abnormalities

Valentina Garibotto, Maria Isabel Vargas, Serge Vulliemoz, and Margitta Seeck

## Introduction

Hypothalamic hamartomas are rare congenital lesions of the hypothalamus, composed of neuronal and glial cells, which can occur sporadically or be associated with other brain lesions or genetic syndromes. They usually present with a drug-resistant epilepsy occurring in the first year of life and they can associate later with endocrinological abnormalities, namely precocious puberty.

The epilepsy can present as multiple seizure types and can be associated with a progressive encephalopathy and developmental decline. The epileptogenicity of the lesion has been confirmed by electrophysiological and imaging observations as well as by the effectiveness of treatments disconnecting the hamartoma on the seizures [1].

2-[$^{18}$F]fluoro-2-deoxy-D-glucose ([$^{18}$F]FDG) PET imaging is often performed in the presurgical evaluation of epilepsy, namely in complex cases with multiple anatomical and electroencephalographic (EEG) abnormalities.

In the literature there is only a limited number of reports describing the [$^{18}$F]FDG PET abnormalities associated with hypothalamic hamartomas.

In ictal conditions, a focal hypermetabolism of the hamartoma was shown [2, 3].

A cortical hypometabolism of variable extent has been described on interictal [$^{18}$F]FDG PET imaging, usually with a lateralization concordant with the anatomical and electroencephalographic lateralization, when present [4–6].

## Case Presentation

A 22 year old patient with drug-resistant focal epilepsy with secondary generalization, severe mental retardation, precocious puberty and behavioral disturbances was evaluated with regard of a radio-surgical treatment.

V. Garibotto (✉)
Division of Nuclear Medicine and Molecular Imaging, Diagnostic Department, University Hospitals of Geneva, Geneva, Switzerland

Faculty of Medicine, University of Geneva, Geneva, Switzerland
e-mail: Valentina.Garibotto@hcuge.ch

M. I. Vargas
Faculty of Medicine, University of Geneva, Geneva, Switzerland

Division of Neuroradiology, Diagnostic Department, University Hospitals of Geneva, Geneva, Switzerland
e-mail: maria.i.vargas@hcuge.ch

S. Vulliemoz · M. Seeck
Faculty of Medicine, University of Geneva, Geneva, Switzerland

Neurology Department, University Hospitals of Geneva, Geneva, Switzerland
e-mail: serge.vulliemoz@hcuge.ch; margitta.seeck@hcuge.ch


A. Varrone et al. (eds.), *Clinical Nuclear Medicine in Neurology*,
https://doi.org/10.1007/978-3-030-83598-9_19

The interictal electroencephalography (EEG) showed a continuous left frontal epileptogenic focus. During the ictal phase a generalized slowing followed by a theta rythm starting in the left frontal region, propagating to the left temporal region and then contralaterally.

## Methods

Magnetic Resonance Imaging (MRI) was performed on a 3 Tesla scanner with a standardized clinical protocol [7].

[$^{18}$F]FDG PET imaging was performed 30 min after injection of 260 MBq of [$^{18}$F]FDG, during the interictal phase, as documented by EEG monitoring and following current procedural guidelines [8].

## Imaging Findings

MRI showed a hypothalamic hamartoma with left lateralization measuring 13 × 10 mm, compressing the mammillary bodies (Fig. 1). The rest of the exam was normal.

[$^{18}$F]FDG PET images showed a left hemispheric cortical hypometabolism, namely in frontal, temporal and parietal regions, associated with a contralateral discrete cerebellar diaschisis (Fig. 2).

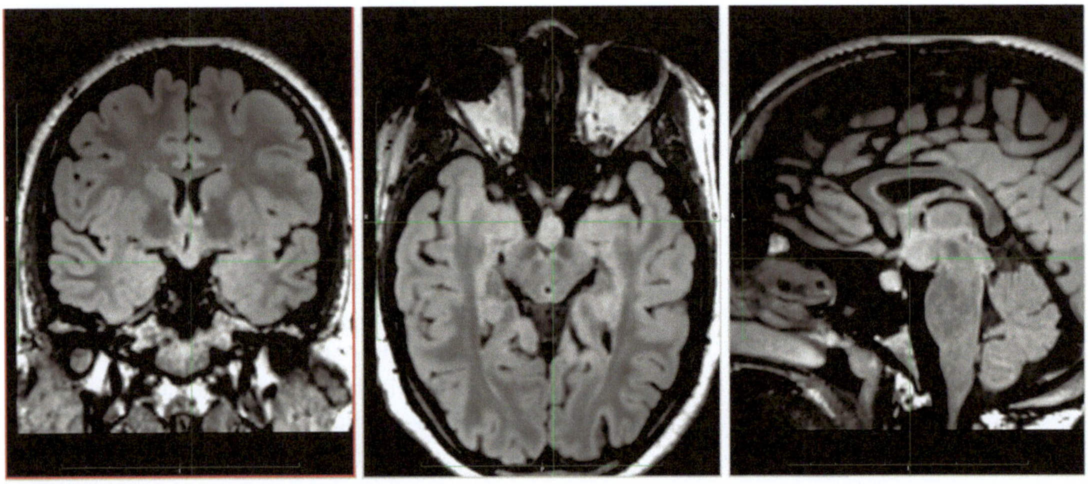

**Fig. 1** Coronal 3D T1 MRI after gadolinium injection showing a left-lateralized hypothalamic hamartoma, as indicated by the crosshair

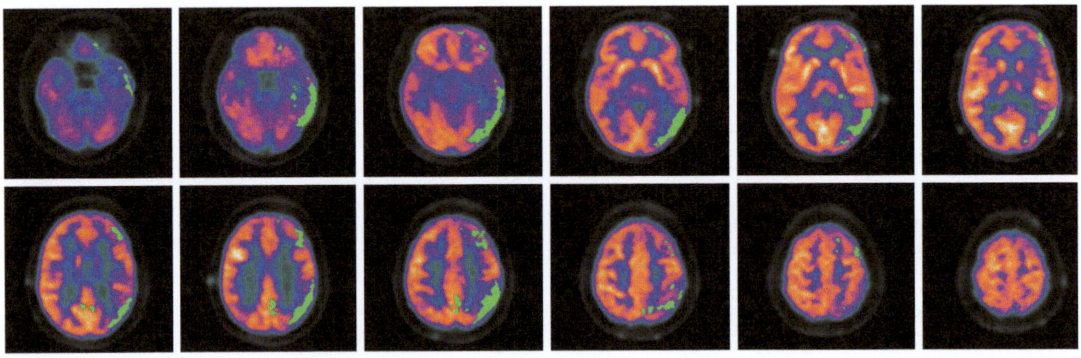

**Fig. 2** Transaxial sections of [$^{18}$F]FDG PET, spatially normalized to a standard template: the green overlay identifies areas below 2.5 standard deviations from the uptake observed in a reference population. A significant hypometabolism was observed in the left temporal, parietal and frontal cortex

## Follow-Up Information

Follow-up evaluation up to 36 months after radiosurgery showed a favorable clinical outcome with a satisfactory control of seizures.

**Take Home Message**

- Thalamic hamartomas can be associated with extensive cortical unilateral hypometabolism corresponding to EEG and anatomic lateralization. Careful correlation of imaging, clinical and electrophysiological data is required to correctly interpret these abnormalities.

## References

1. Ferrand-Sorbets S, Fohlen M, Delalande O, Zuber K, Bulteau C, Levy M, Chamard P, Taussig D, Dorison N, Bekaert O, et al. Seizure outcome and prognostic factors for surgical management of hypothalamic hamartomas in children. Seizure. 2020;75:28–33.
2. Palmini A, Van Paesschen W, Dupont P, Van Laere K, Van Driel G. Status gelasticus after temporal lobectomy: ictal FDG-PET findings and the question of dual pathology involving hypothalamic hamartomas. Epilepsia. 2005;46(8):1313–6.
3. Shahar E, Goldsher D, Genizi J, Ravid S, Keidar Z. Intractable gelastic seizures during infancy: ictal positron emission tomography (PET) demonstrating epileptiform activity within the hypothalamic hamartoma. J Child Neurol. 2008;23(2):235–9.
4. Meyer MA. Temporal lobe Hypometabolism ipsilateral to a hypothalamic mass. Relationship to gelastic seizures. Clin Positron Imaging. 2000;3(2):75–7.
5. Ryvlin P, Ravier C, Bouvard S, Mauguire F, Le Bars D, Arzimanoglou A, Petit J, Kahane P. Positron emission tomography in epileptogenic hypothalamic hamartomas. Epileptic Disord. 2003;5(4):219–27.
6. Wagner K, Schulze-Bonhage A, Urbach H, Trippel M, Spehl TS, Buschmann F, Metternich B, Ofer I, Meyer PT, Frings L. Reduced glucose metabolism in neocortical network nodes remote from hypothalamic hamartomas reflects cognitive impairment. Epilepsia. 2017;58(Suppl 2):41–9.
7. Fitsiori A, Hiremath SB, Boto J, Garibotto V, Vargas MI. Morphological and advanced imaging of epilepsy: beyond the basics. Children (Basel). 2019;6(3):43.
8. Varrone A, Asenbaum S, Vander Borght T, Booij J, Nobili F, Nagren K, Darcourt J, Kapucu OL, Tatsch K, Bartenstein P, et al. EANM procedure guidelines for PET brain imaging using [18F]FDG, version 2. Eur J Nucl Med Mol Imaging. 2009;36(12):2103–10.

# Case 20: Autoimmune Encephalitis with Unusual Antibodies

Javier Arbizu and Juan Jose Rosales

## Case Summary

A 65-year-old male referred a recent episode of acute memory loss lasted 30–60 min. It consisted of inability of recording new information and difficulty in recalling events and conversations from the previous days. He did not reflect clear trigger factors, although he suffered from diabetes type 2 and hypertension, and had prior history of acute myocardium infarct with cardiorespiratory arrest 10 years ago. He was evaluated in a local hospital where the brain CT and MRI scans were normal, without any brain bleeding or ischemic brain infarct, and laboratory investigations only showed a high serum creatine kinase level (323 U/L). He totally recovered after several hours and was diagnosed of transient global amnesia.

In the last 2 weeks before admission in our center, he referred isolated episodes of sweating, chills, and piloerection that increased in frequency up to 14 times a day, and his relatives described occasional drowsiness and difficulty to recognize people or remember recent events.

The physical and neurological examinations were normal, without cognitive loss or motor deficits. The routine laboratory test was also within the normal limits, and the electroencephalogram showed normal wave pattern. Nevertheless, the patient was admitted in our hospital for further evaluation.

## Images/Findings

In an attempt to elucidate the origin of these episodes, different complementary tests including multimodal imaging, lumbar puncture, serology, 24 h video electroencephalogram (video-EEG) monitoring among others were requested.

The brain MRI reflected a bilateral amygdalo-hippocampal enlargement, particularly in the right medial temporal, which exhibited a hyperintensity on T2-weighted fluid-attenuated inversion recovery (FLAIR) sequences, without any additional pathological findings (Fig. 1). The differential diagnosis was established between a low-grade glioma of the right medial temporal lobe, a developing encephalitis (limbic or herpetic), or related to epileptic seizures.

The whole-body PET-CT using [$^{18}$F]fluorodeoxiglucose (FDG-PET) showed mild bilateral pleural effusion and diffuse increased prostate uptake (maximum Standard Uptake Value: 4.8) suggesting prostatitis, but without evidence of any systemic malignant neoplasm (Fig. 2).

In the brain FDG-PET scan, there was a marked hypermetabolism in the right anterior medial temporal cortex (Fig. 3), which matched with the

J. Arbizu (✉) · J. J. Rosales
Department of Nuclear Medicine, Clinica Universidad de Navarra, University of Navarra, Pamplona, Spain
e-mail: jarbizu@unav.es


A. Varrone et al. (eds.), *Clinical Nuclear Medicine in Neurology*,
https://doi.org/10.1007/978-3-030-83598-9_20

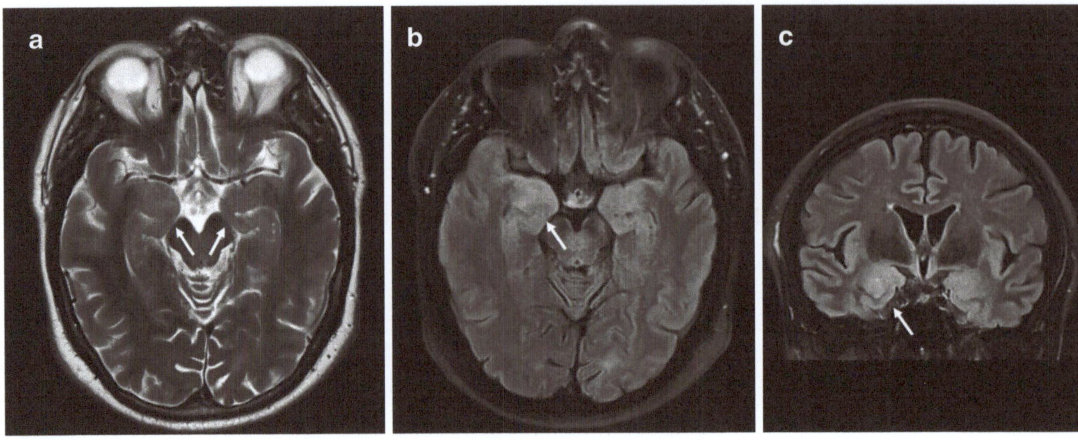


**Fig. 1** Axial slices of T2-weighted and T2-weighted FLAIR brain MRI sequences (**a**, **b**) and T2-weighted FLAIR coronal slice. There was a bilateral amygdalo-hippocampal enlargement (white arrows in **a**), with marked hyperintensity in right side (white arrow in **b** and **c**)

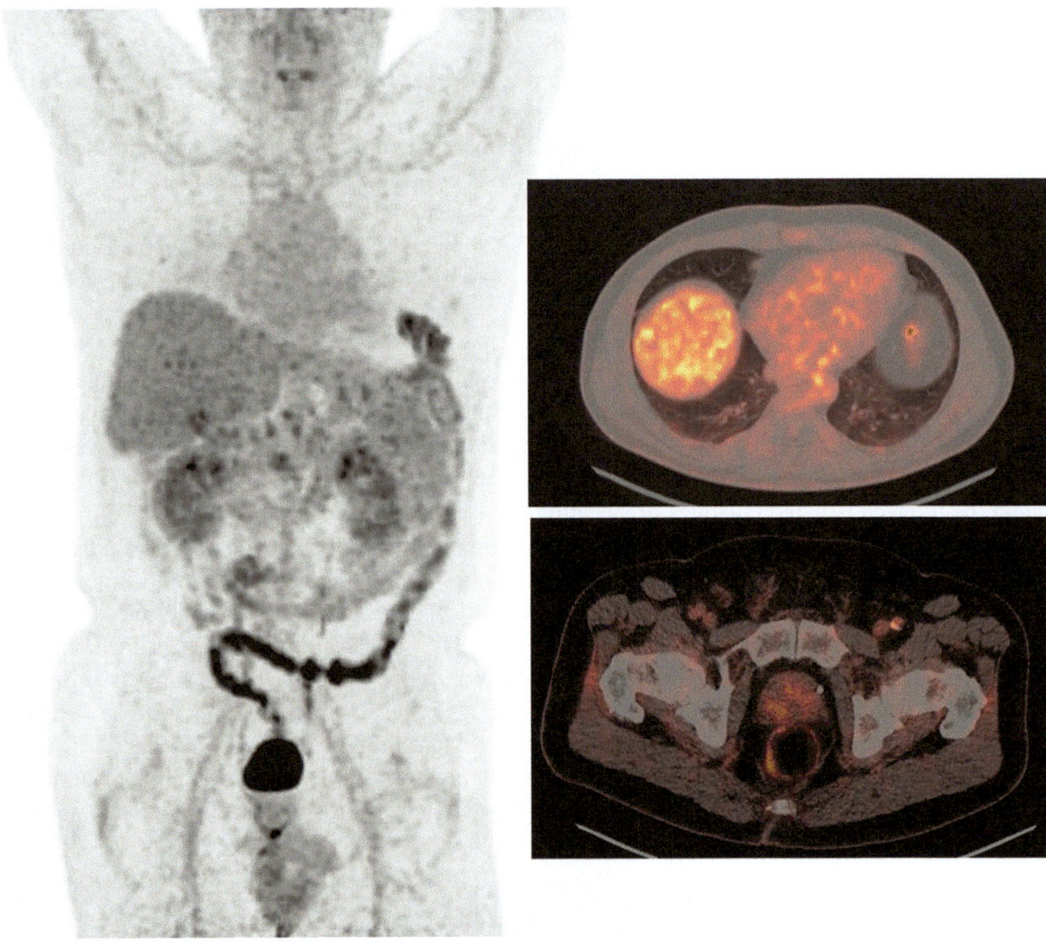

**Fig. 2** Whole-body FDG-PET without evidence of systemic neoplasm. There was a diffuse increase of bowel activity (particularly in the colon) due to inflammation related to antidiabetic treatment (metformin). On the PT/CT fusion axial slices, it can be seen mild lung and prostate inflammatory uptake

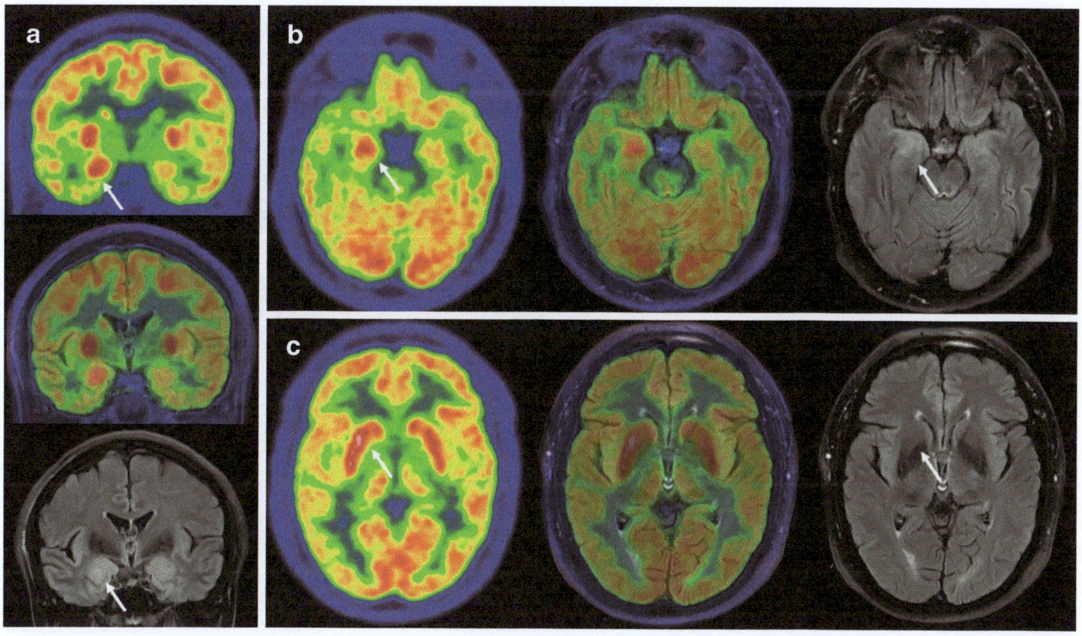


**Fig. 3** [[18]F]FDG-PET images. Coronal (**a**) and axial (**b**, **c**) slices of PET, fused PET/MRI and MRI showing an increased metabolic activity in the right medial temporal lobe that matches the MRI hyperintensity (white arrows in **a** and **b**)

amygdalo-hypoccampal hyperintensity described in the $T_2$-FLAIR MRI sequences (Fig. 3). Interestingly, the 3D statistical surface projections obtained after comparing with a normal database reflected a bilateral significant increased activity of the medial temporal lobes (Fig. 4). In addition, the right basal ganglia presented an increased metabolism (Figs. 3 and 4). All these findings suggested the diagnosis of limbic encephalitis.

The analysis of cerebrospinal fluid (CSF) revealed an increase of cellularity (7 cells/μL), increased glucose (90 mg/dL), and proteins (63 mg/dL). On the other hand, the serology for syphilis, herpes virus (1–2 and 6), and HIV testing in serum and CSF were negative.

Video-EEG displayed normal interictal activity with right medial temporal epileptic activity during the two recorded episodes of chills and piloerection.

With a clinical suspicion of limbic encephalitis, the patient started treatment with intravenous immunoglobulin (0.4 g/kg/day) and methylprednisolone (1 g/day) during 5 days with good tolerance and clinical improvement. Moreover, the patient required supplementary antiepileptic treatment.

Screening for common anti-neuropil antibodies (Hu, Yo, Ri, Tr, CV2, anphiphysin, MA2, SOX1) was negative. However, CASPR2 neuronal surface antibodies were detected in serum and CSF.

Two additional cycles of immunoglobulins were administered 1 and 3 months after patient hospital discharge. However, he presented early recurrence of epileptic seizures after immunoglobulin administration. Consequently, an additional fourth cycle of immunoglobulin was administered in conjunction with rituximab (375 mg/m$^2$) with complete remission of symptoms. The patient remains asymptomatic after 3 years of follow-up without active treatment.

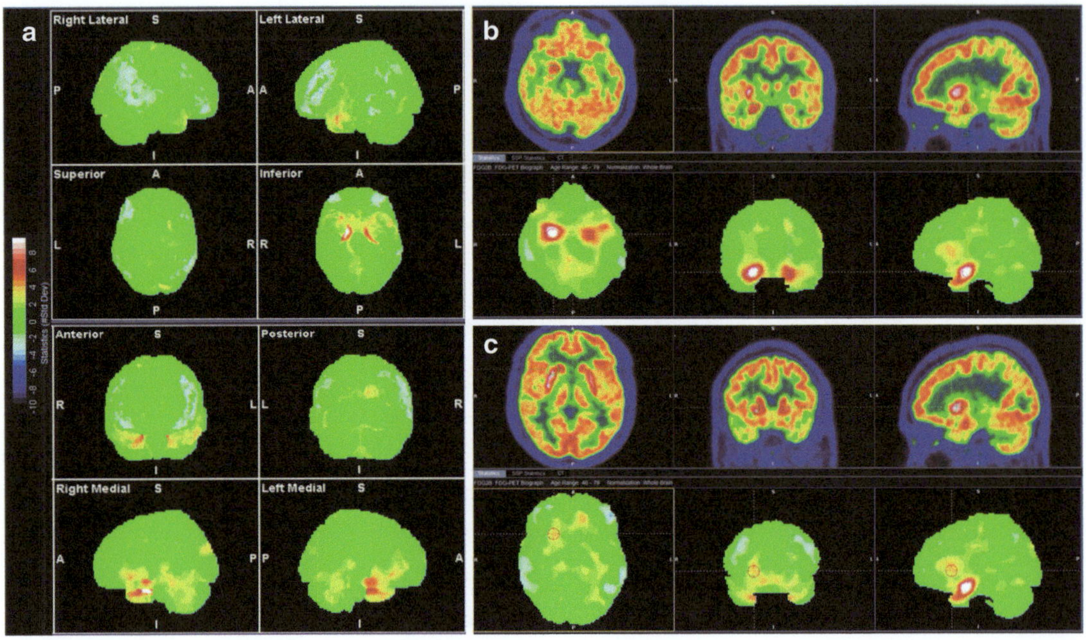


**Fig. 4** [[18]F]FDG-PET stereotactic surface projections (Syngo.via Database Comparison, Siemens) (**a**) revealed a significant bilateral hypermetabolism in medial temporal lobes. The axial, coronal, and sagittal images and statistical maps (**b**) show in detail the bilateral increases in the medial temporal lobe (more significant in the right side, red circle). Interestingly, the right putamen (**c**) presented an increased metabolism, which was only statistically significant in the anterior part (red circle)

## Diagnosis

Autoimmune limbic encephalitis mediated by CASPR 2 antibodies.

## Discussion

Autoimmune encephalitis (AE) is an inflammatory brain disorder associated with neurologic dysfunction and is frequently a challenging clinical diagnosis as it mimics other conditions without treatment like Alzheimer's disease or Creutzfeldt–Jakob disease. AE limbic encephalitis (LE) is a specific type of AE in which inflammation affects predominantly the medial temporal lobes. LE may present with memory impairment, hallucinations, anxiety, irritability, depression, seizures, and sleep alterations [1]. The pathogenesis of AE is related to the presence of autoantibodies against intracellular antigens (Hu, Ma2, GAD), synaptic receptors (NMDA receptor, AMPA receptor, GABA receptor, mGluR5, Dopamine receptor), ion channels, and other cell-surface proteins (LGI-1, CASPR2, DPPX; MOG, AQP4, GQ1b) [1, 2]. The most frequent antibody related to LE is LGI-1 and other like CASPR2 are less common [3].

Antibodies against CASPR2 are directed to the extracellular domain and target inhibitory interneurons in the hippocampus. Anti-CASPR2-mediated disease has a strong predominance in men (90%) with an age at onset around 60–70 years. Clinical presentation is heterogeneous and can include cerebral symptoms (cognition, epilepsy), cerebellar symptoms, peripheral nerve hyperexcitability, autonomic dysfunction, insomnia, neuropathic pain, and weight loss. The disease usually has a more indolent course and progression over 1 year; hence, it can mimic neurodegenerative disorders, especially in patients with cognitive decline [4].

First-line treatment of LE include steroids, intravenous immunoglobulin, or a combination of both. Additionally, some patients require second-line treatments such as rituximab and/or cyclophosphamide [5]. Therefore, LE is a treatable condition with total clinical recovery, but treatment is often delayed due to the lack of specific symptoms and the time it takes to obtain the result of the autoantibodies analysis. Recently, a clinical approach was proposed to treat subjects with a high clinical suspicion of AE, including LE, potentially leading to better outcomes [2].

Unfortunately, routine laboratory test can be normal and mild cell counts or protein levels can be detected in CSF at the disease onset. EEG results are usually nonspecific, but sometimes epileptic or slow wave activity involving the temporal lobes can be seen [1, 2]. CASPR2 antibodies can be detected by brain tissue immunohistochemistry and can be specifically confirmed with a cell-based assay.

Typical brain MRI findings in AE include hyperintense signal on T2-weighted fluid-attenuated inversion recovery sequences highly restricted to one or both medial temporal lobes (limbic encephalitis), or in multifocal areas involving gray matter, white matter, or both compatible with demyelination or inflammation. However, these findings cannot be present at disease onset or results unspecific as they may also appear in other conditions (i.e., Creutzfeldt–Jakob disease, glioma).

[$^{18}$F]FDG PET imaging can show medial temporal lobe hypermetabolism even in the absence of abnormalities in the brain MRI [2, 3, 6]. Therefore, patients with AE may benefit from prompt diagnosis when brain FDG-PET is added to the traditional complementary tests. At this respect, it is important to note the usefulness of voxel-based analysis of FDG-PET images in defining specific patterns and helping the clinical diagnosis of AE [7]. Whole-body [$^{18}$F]FDG PET/CT can also contribute to exclude potential systemic malignancies, especially in patients with Morvan syndrome with anti CASPR2 antibodies, which has been associated with the presence of thymoma up to 40% [1].

## Conclusions

[$^{18}$F]FDG PET can reveal specific metabolic patterns depending on the subtype of autoimmune encephalitis that could help to reach an early clinical diagnosis and start the treatment. Even though its use is not directly included in clinical diagnostic guidelines, FDG-PET is currently accepted to fulfill the imaging criteria when brain MRI appears normal [2].

## References


1. Dalmau J, Graus F. Antibody-mediated encephalitis. N Engl J Med. 2018;378:840–51.
2. Graus F, Titulaer MJ, Balu R, Benseler S, Bien CG, Cellucci T, et al. A clinical approach to diagnosis of autoimmune encephalitis. Lancet Neurol. 2016;15:391–404.
3. Probasco JC, Solnes L, Nalluri A, Cohen J, Jones KM, Zan E, et al. Abnormal brain metabolism on FDG-PET/CT is a common early finding in autoimmune encephalitis. Neurol Neuroimmunol Neuroinflamm. 2017;4:e352.
4. Van Sonderen A, Petit-Pedrol M, Dalmau J, Titulaer MJ. The value of LGI1, Caspr2 and voltage-gated potassium channel antibodies in encephalitis. Nat Rev Neurol. 2017;13:290–301.
5. Liu R, Zhang M, Liu L, Chen G, Hou Y, Wang M, et al. Neuronal surface antibody syndrome: a review of the characteristics of the disease and its association with autoantibodies. Neuroimmunomodulation. 2020;27:1–8.
6. Morbelli S, Arbizu J, Booij J, Chen MK, Chetelat G, Cross DJ, et al. The need of standardization and of large clinical studies in an emerging indication of [18F]FDG PET: the autoimmune encephalitis. Eur J Nucl Med Mol Imaging. 2017;44:353–7.
7. Moreno-Ajona D, Prieto E, Grisanti F, Esparragosa I, Sánchez Orduz L, Gállego Pérez-Larraya J, et al. 18F-FDG-PET imaging patterns in autoimmune encephalitis: impact of image analysis on the results. Diagnostics (Basel). 2020;10(6):e356.

# Case 21: Psychiatric Presentation of Anti-*N*-Methyl-D-Aspartate Receptor (NMDAR) Limbic Encephalitis

Tatiana Horowitz, Elsa Kaphan, and Eric Guedj

## Case Summary

A 29-year-old woman with personal history of depressive disorder since the age of 17 years was admitted for major depression and catatonia. She had lowered her antidepressant treatments recently since she expressed the desire of pregnancy. Depressive symptoms worsened, and a catatonic syndrome appeared with episodes of agitation and hallucinations. An organic etiology was suspected since antipsychotic and antidepressant drugs had no effect. Brain MRI was negative, cerebrospinal fluid cell count and protein were normal, but anti-NMDAR antibodies were identified. Brain [$^{18}$F]FDG PET-CT showed a limbic encephalitis pattern, and whole-body PET-CT did not reveal any tumor. Plasmapheresis along with corticosteroids was first attempted. She recovered after second-line rituximab immunotherapy.

Brain PET in a 29-year-old woman with rapidly progressive psychiatric symptoms and normal MRI (Fig. 1).

## Epidemiology

- Limbic encephalitis (LE) is a rare condition where limbic areas are affected by an autoimmune antibody-mediated process.
- NMDAR type is the most frequent cause of LE and affects more often women (sex ratio 4:1).

## Pathology

- Antibodies can target cell membrane antigens such as NMDAR or intracellular antigens.
- Can be paraneoplastic or not.
- NMDAR type is especially associated with tumors such as ovarian teratoma.

## Clinical Findings

- Lesions of limbic areas cause subacute memory deficit, seizures, autonomic dysfunction, psychiatric symptoms.
- Psychiatric forms of LE are often more difficult to diagnose.

T. Horowitz · E. Guedj (✉)
CERIMED, Nuclear Medicine Department, Timone Hospital, Aix Marseille Univ, APHM, CNRS, Centrale Marseille, Institut Fresnel, Marseille, France
e-mail: eric.guedj@univ-amu.fr

E. Kaphan
Aix Marseille Univ, APHM, Hôpital de la Timone, Pôle de Neurosciences Cliniques, Service de Neurologie, Marseille, France


A. Varrone et al. (eds.), *Clinical Nuclear Medicine in Neurology*,
https://doi.org/10.1007/978-3-030-83598-9_21

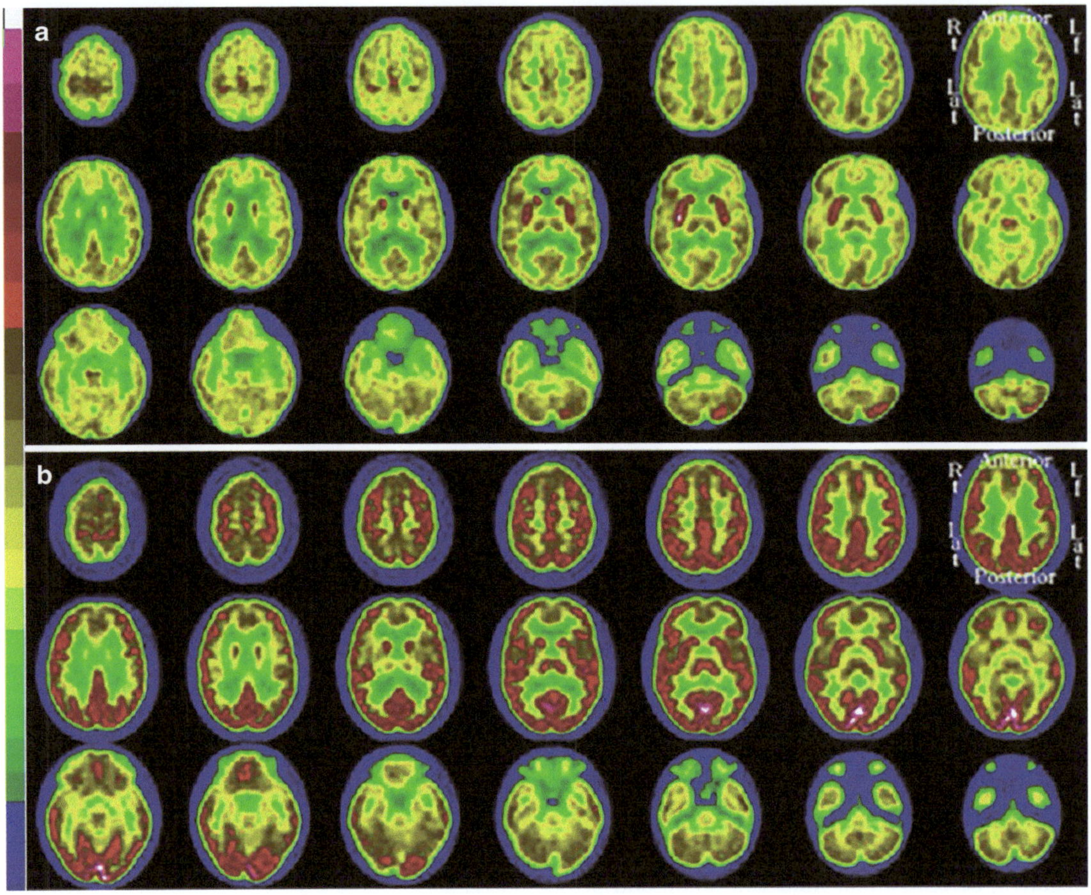


**Fig. 1** (**a**) Axial [$^{18}$F]FDG PET-CT slices at onset of symptoms showing diffuse brain hypometabolism including marked medial temporal hypometabolism, and relative hypermetabolism of striata, mesencephalon and left cerebellar hemisphere, suggestive of limbic encephalitis. (**b**) Axial [$^{18}$F]FDG PET-CT slices after immunotherapy showing normalization of brain metabolism

## Treatment

- Immunotherapy and tumor surgery when present.
- About 80% improvement after immunotherapy in NMDAR type.
- Early treatment is a predictor of good outcome.

## Imaging Findings

- MRI classically shows abnormalities of medial temporal regions, but can be often normal.
- Typical patterns are described in [$^{18}$F]FDG PET: widespread cortical hypometabolism with striatal ± medial temporal hypermetabolism.

**Take-Home Message**

- [$^{18}$F]FDG PET-CT is an essential tool for the early diagnose and follow-up of LE and is particularly helpful when MRI is negative.

## Further Reading

Baumgartner A, Rauer S, Mader I, et al. Cerebral FDG-PET and MRI findings in autoimmune limbic encephalitis: correlation with autoantibody types. J Neurol. 2013;260:2744–53.

Bordonne M, Chawki MB, Doyen M, et al. Brain (18)F-FDG PET for the diagnosis of autoimmune encephalitis: a systematic review and a meta-analysis. Eur J Nucl Med Mol Imaging. 2021. https://doi.org/10.1007/s00259-021-05299-y.

Leypoldt F, Buchert R, Kleiter I, et al. Fluorodeoxyglucose positron emission tomography in anti-N-methyl-D-aspartate receptor encephalitis: distinct pattern of disease. J Neurol Neurosurg Psychiatry. 2012;83:681–6.

# Case 22: Hashimoto Encephalitis

Tatiana Horowitz, Elsa Kaphan, and Eric Guedj

**Case Summary** A 69-year-old woman was admitted in intensive care unit for movement disorders and altered level of consciousness up to coma. The clinical presentation started 4 months prior to admission to the acute care unit with intermittent tremors and episodes of stupor. Status epilepticus was then suspected, but EEGs were unconclusive. Brain MRI was normal. She had a previous history of left thyroidectomy for goiter and thyroiditis at the age of 39 years. Blood test revealed isolated elevated titers of antithyroid peroxidase. Lumbar puncture was normal. She underwent a whole-body PET-CT, showing increased [$^{18}$F]FDG uptake in thyroid goiter. The decision was made to do a thyroidectomy, but surgeons did not want to proceed surgery until she was out of the coma, and corticosteroid could not be started because a thyroid lymphoma was suspected. Brain [$^{18}$F]FDG PET-CT contributed to the diagnosis of encephalitis, convincing surgeons to do thyroidectomy in this context. Anatomopathological analysis confirmed thyroiditis and excluded lymphoma. She fully recovered with combined corticosteroid therapy.

PET in a 69-year-old woman with movement disorders, coma, and history of goiter (Figs. 1, 2 and 3).

## Epidemiology

- Rare, controversial encephalopathy associated with Hashimoto thyroiditis.
- Affects more often women.

## Clinical Features

- Nonspecific encephalitis symptoms: movement disorders, seizures, psychiatric manifestations, confusion, coma, cognitive impairment, focal deficits.
- Associated with Hashimoto thyroiditis.

## Pathology

- Unknown pathophysiology.
- Elevated titers of antithyroid peroxidase or antithyroglobulin antibodies in serum.
- Thyroid function usually normal.

T. Horowitz · E. Guedj (✉)
CERIMED, Nuclear Medicine Department, Aix Marseille Univ, APHM, CNRS, Centrale Marseille, Institut Fresnel, Timone Hospital, Marseille, France
e-mail: eric.guedj@univ-amu.fr

E. Kaphan
Service de Neurologie, Aix Marseille Univ, APHM, Hôpital de la Timone, Pôle de Neurosciences Cliniques, Marseille, France



A. Varrone et al. (eds.), *Clinical Nuclear Medicine in Neurology*,
https://doi.org/10.1007/978-3-030-83598-9_22

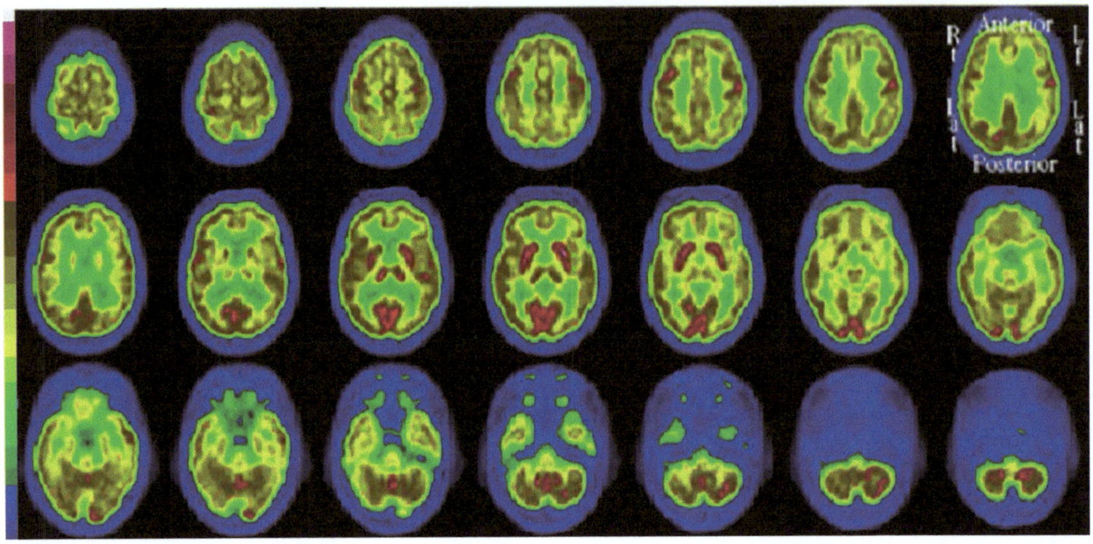


**Fig. 1** Axial [18F]FDG PET-CT slices at onset of symptoms showing diffuse brain hypometabolism and striatal hypermetabolism, suggestive of encephalitis

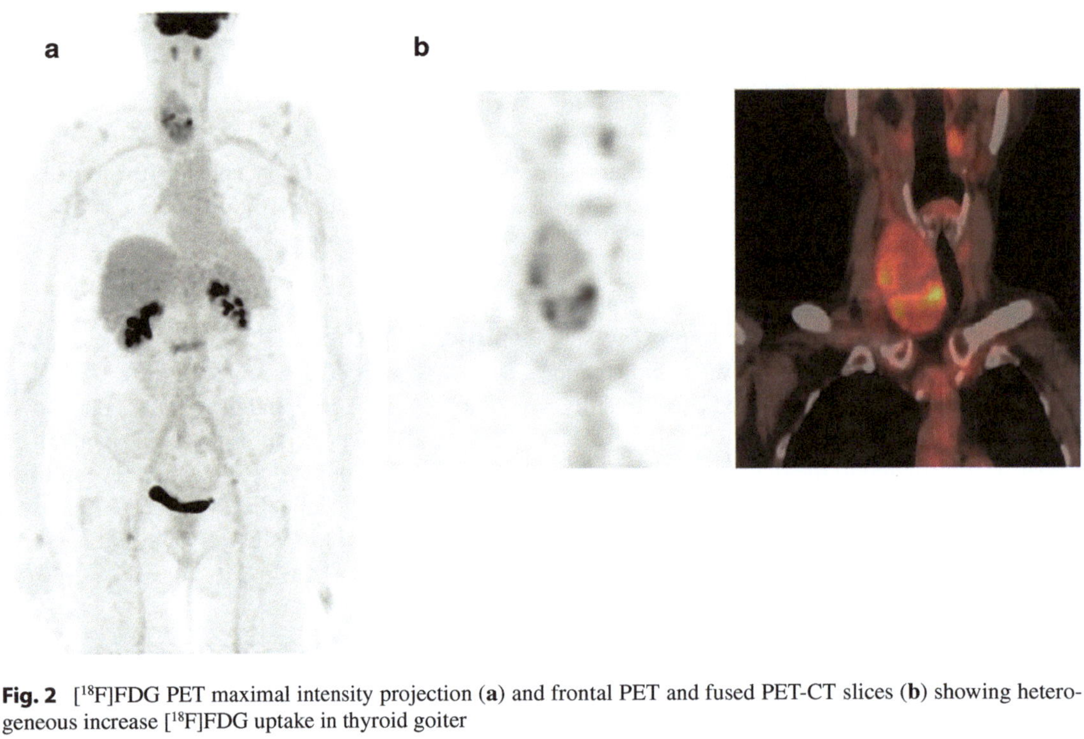


**Fig. 2** [18F]FDG PET maximal intensity projection (**a**) and frontal PET and fused PET-CT slices (**b**) showing heterogeneous increase [18F]FDG uptake in thyroid goiter

## Clinical Management

- Steroid response in about half of patients.
- Plasma exchange or intravenous immunoglobulin can be effective.

## Imaging Findings

- MRI can show white matter hyperintensities, or limbic-encephalitis-like manifestations with temporal FLAIR hypersignal, but remains normal in most cases.

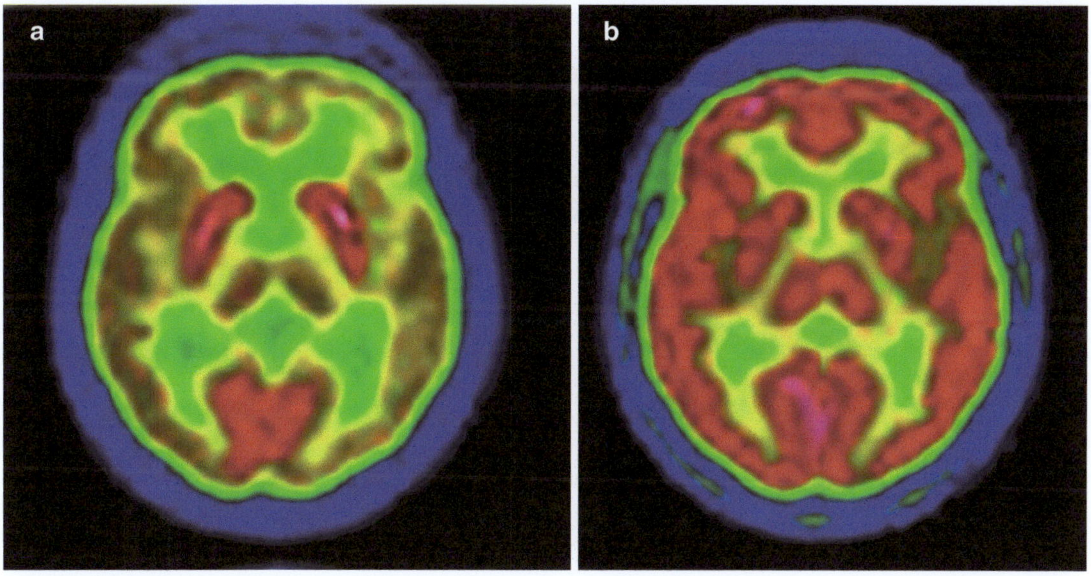


**Fig. 3** Axial [$^{18}$F]FDG PET-CT slice before (**a**) and after thyroidectomy and corticosteroid therapy (**b**) showing normalization of brain metabolism

- [$^{18}$F]FDG brain PET-CT usually show signs of encephalitis with diffuse brain hypometabolism and striatal ± medial temporal hypermetabolism.

**Take-Home Message**

- Hashimoto encephalopathy can present as encephalitis on brain [$^{18}$F]FDG PET images.

## Further Reading

Nagano M, Kobayashi K, Yamada-Otani M, Kuzuya A, Matsumoto R, Oita J, Yoneda M, Ikeda A, Takahashi R. Hashimoto's encephalopathy presenting with smoldering limbic encephalitis. Intern Med. 2019;58(8):1167–72. Epub 2019 Apr 15. PMID: 30982805; PMCID: PMC6522399. https://doi.org/10.2169/internalmedicine.1289-18.

Zhou JY, Xu B, Lopes J, Blamoun J, Li L. Hashimoto encephalopathy: literature review. Acta Neurol Scand. 2017;135(3):285–90. Epub 2016 Jun 20. https://doi.org/10.1111/ane.12618.

# Section III

# Nuclear Medicine Cases of Brain Tumors

# Case 23: Pseudoresponse in Glioblastoma

Ian Law, Jonathan F. Carlsen, and Benedikte Hasselbalch

## Patient

- A 54-year-old man with glioblastoma, IDH wt, in left parietal lobe. Previously treated with resection and concomitant radiation chemotherapy (temozolomide). First recurrence close to the motor cortex on the left side. Resection is declined.

## Background

- Response assessment in glioma using conventional MRI is based on the measurement of contrast enhancement reflecting a disrupted blood brain barrier (BBB).
- Pseudoresponse is a condition where contrast enhancement is falsely reduced due to changes in vascular permeability independent of antitumor effects resulting in high response rates (~50%) without significant changes in overall survival.
- Pseudoresponse is found with antiangiogenic therapy, e.g., bevacizumab, targeting vascular endothelial growth factor (VEGF) pro-angiogenic signaling pathways and is expressed by a vascular normalization and decreased BBB permeability independent of an antitumor effect.
- As blood supply to the glioma can no longer be sustained by neovascularization, antiangiogenic treatment induces a selection pressure that may promote glioma cell clones with a diffusely infiltrative growth pattern ("gliomatosis"), meeting metabolic demands by co-opting existing vasculature independent of angiogenesis.
- T2 FLAIR MRI signal changes can be used in response assessment, but may be challenged by treatment-related damage derived from surgery, irradiation, and chemotherapy.
- Diffusion weighted imaging (DWI) and apparent diffusion coefficient (ADC) MRI of water diffusion restriction as a marker of increased cellularity in glioma have been suggested as an adjunct in the identification of pseudoresponse. This, however, should be regarded as a research area since the literature is conflicting.
- Amino acid PET tracers are transported into glioma by the L-amino transporter (LAT) independent of a blood–brain barrier disruption and can identify active tumor tissue in patients with misclassified treatment response on conventional MRI (Figs. 1, 2, and 3).

I. Law (✉)
Department of Clinical Physiology, Nuclear Medicine and PET, University of Copenhagen, Copenhagen, Denmark
e-mail: ian.law@regionh.dk

J. F. Carlsen
Department of Diagnostic Radiology, University of Copenhagen, Copenhagen, Denmark

B. Hasselbalch
Department of Oncology, Rigshospitalet, University of Copenhagen, Copenhagen, Denmark


A. Varrone et al. (eds.), *Clinical Nuclear Medicine in Neurology*,
https://doi.org/10.1007/978-3-030-83598-9_23

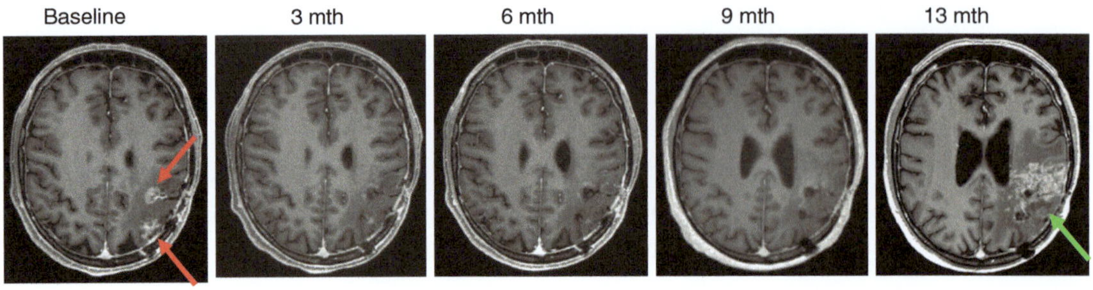


**Fig. 1** T1 postcontrast MRI before onset of second-line combined bevacizumab and lomustine treatment and at follow-up scans 3, 6, and 9 months after which the treatment was changed to Irinotecan monotherapy. Treatment response according to the RANO criteria is reported with regression of contrast-enhancing tumor (red arrows) and with discrete and stable unmeasurable contrast-enhancing tumor before withdrawal of antiangiogenic treatment after 9 months. The 13 months scan show a typical rebound phenomenon demasking active tumor tissue in the region (green arrow). Active treatment was withdrawn and the patient referred to the palliative care

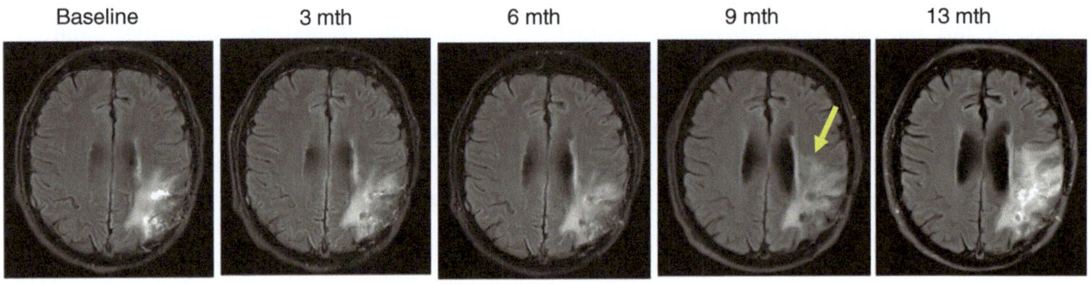


**Fig. 2** T2 FLAIR MRI scans at the same positions as in Fig. 1 showing initially stable signal changes with slight signal increase at 9 months (yellow arrow). Any tumor-related progression in FLAIR signal may be masked by persistent treatment related changes around the cavity

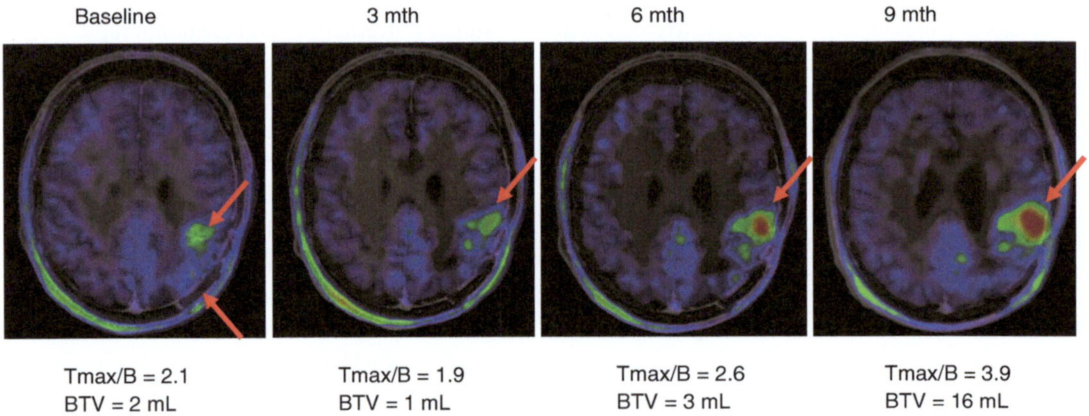


**Fig. 3** PET scans using the amino acid analog tracer O-(2-[$^{18}$F]fluoroethyl)-L-tyrosine ([$^{18}$F]FET) fused to T1 postcontrast MRI at the same positions and follow-up times as in Figs. 1 and 2. Only the most anterior lesion contrast enhancement is active (red arrows), indicating treatment damage in the posterior lesion. After an initial response, a continuous increase in metabolic activity (Tmax/B) and biological tumor volume (BTV, red arrow) is identified despite stable conditions on MRI. This is in accordance with a diagnosis of pseudoresponse

## Occurrence

- In glioblastoma patients up to 1/3 treated with antiangiogenic therapy and 1/10 with conventional concomitant radio-chemotherapy may progress with non-contrast enhancement on conventional MRI.

## Imaging Findings

- Apparent treatment response with a reduction in contrast-enhancing tumor om MRI.
- Stable or slowly progressing diffuse or circumscribed T2 FLAIR MRI signal hyperintensity.
- Increased uptake using amino acid PET tracers usually corresponding to the T2 FLAIR signal.
- Rebound in contrast enhancement following withdrawal of antiangiogenic treatment.

## Clinical Management

- Tumor progression is an expression of treatment failure and alternative options will be considered including resection, irradiation, chemotherapy, or palliative care.

**Take-Home Message**
- Consider using amino acid PET imaging to assess treatment response in antiangiogenic therapy, particularly in patients with uncertainties in conventional MRI and clinical progression.
- The presence of biologically active glioma tissue is supported by persistent or increasing uptake on sequential amino acid PET imaging.
- Usually Tmax/B values above 2.0 is indicative of active tumor.

## Further Reading

Aquino D, Gioppo A, Finocchiaro G, Bruzzone MG, Cuccarini V. MRI in glioma immunotherapy: evidence, pitfalls, and perspectives. J Immunol Res. 2017;2017:5813951.

Auer TA, Breit HC, Marini F, et al. Evaluation of the apparent diffusion coefficient in patients with recurrent glioblastoma under treatment with bevacizumab with radiographic pseudoresponse. J Neuroradiol. 2019;46:36–43.

Hutterer M, Nowosielski M, Putzer D, et al. O-(2-18F-fluoroethyl)-L-tyrosine PET predicts failure of antiangiogenic treatment in patients with recurrent high-grade glioma. J Nucl Med. 2011;52:856–64.

Nowosielski M, Ellingson BM, Chinot OL, et al. Radiologic progression of glioblastoma under therapy-an exploratory analysis of AVAglio. Neuro Oncol. 2018;20:557–66.

# Case 24: Progressive Glioma

Ian Law, Jonathan F. Carlsen,
and Benedikte Hasselbalch

## Patient

- A 49-year-old man with anaplastic oligodendroglioma, WHO grade III, IDH mut in the left parietooccipital region treated with previous resection followed by proton therapy and chemotherapy with procarbazine, lomustine, and vincristine (PCV).
- MRI (Fig. 1, baseline) without concurrent chemotherapy showed cloudy, speckled new non-measurable contrast enhancement, while older speckles dissolved, and stable non-contrast-enhancing signal changes (Fig. 2) compared to MRI 3 and 6 months previously. No clinical progression was reported. The presence of active tumor tissue was uncertain, and the patient was referred to O-(2-[$^{18}$F]fluoroethyl)-L-tyrosine ([$^{18}$F]FET) PET scan for further evaluation.
- Based on increased metabolic activity, treatment with temozolomide was initiated (Fig. 3).
- In clinical follow-up, the patient experienced slight right-sided motor weakness (Figs. 4 and 5). Although follow-up MRI (Fig. 1, 12 months) showed progression of non-contrast-enhancing signal changes, the changing pattern of speckled new and dissolving old non-measurable contrast enhancement persisted. An additional [$^{18}$F]FET PET scan was performed for further confirmation, indicating treatment failure with marked progression and distant spread to the cerebellar vermis (Fig. 6).
- Therapy was changed to antiangiogenic therapy (bevacizumab) and irinotecan.

## Background

- Treatment options at progression are limited for patients with glioma. Thus, accuracy in the definition of progression is essential.
- Definition of progression is based on Response Assessment in Neuro-oncology (RANO) criteria and rests primarily on conventional MRI and measurements of contrast enhancement, reflecting a disrupted blood–brain barrier.
- Clinically asymptomatic, newly detected, non-measurable speckled contrast-enhancing

I. Law (✉)
Department of Clinical Physiology, Nuclear Medicine and PET, University of Copenhagen, Copenhagen, Denmark
e-mail: ian.law@regionh.dk

J. F. Carlsen
Department of Diagnostic Radiology, University of Copenhagen, Copenhagen, Denmark

B. Hasselbalch
Department of Oncology, Rigshospitalet, University of Copenhagen, Copenhagen, Denmark



A. Varrone et al. (eds.), *Clinical Nuclear Medicine in Neurology*,
https://doi.org/10.1007/978-3-030-83598-9_24

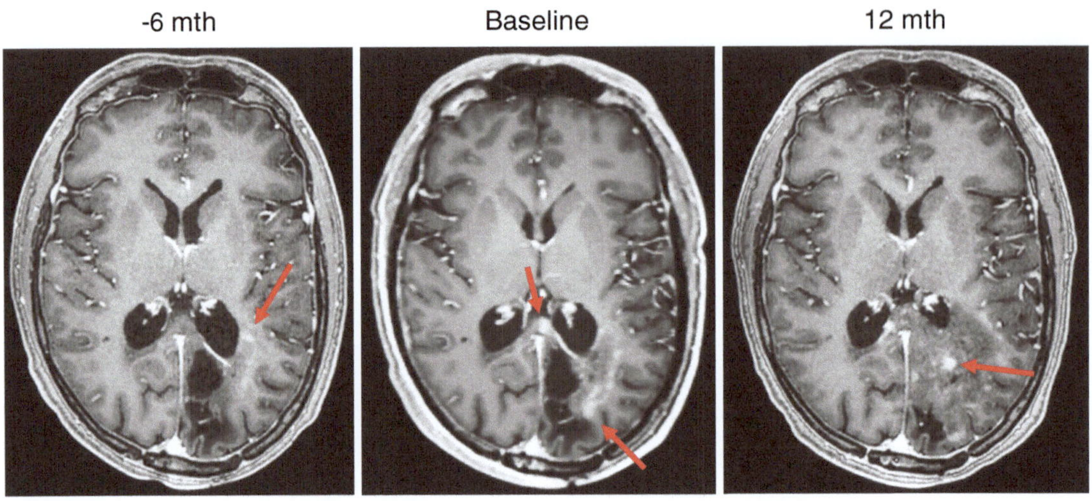


**Fig. 1** T1 postcontrast MRI at 6 months prior, at untreated baseline, and at follow-up 12 months after temozolomide, showing changing patterns of speckled new and dissolving old non-measurable contrast enhancement (red arrows) none of which can satisfy the RANO criteria for progressive disease (>10 × 10 mm)

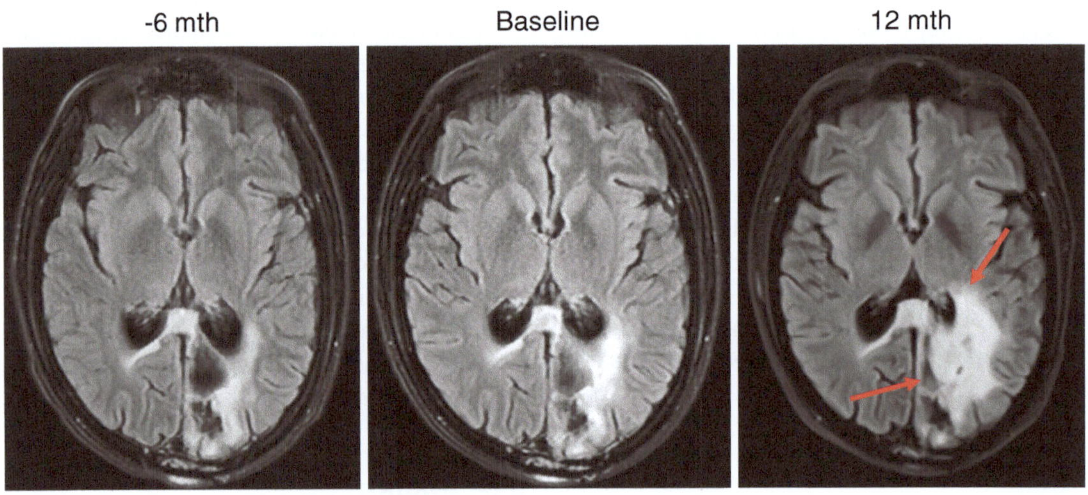


**Fig. 2** T2 FLAIR MRI at the same positions as in Fig. 1. Baseline showed stable non-contrast-enhancing signal changes compared to 6 months previously, while there was progression at 12 months at the medial border and increasing encroachment of the occipital horn of the left ventricle (red arrows)

lesions appear relatively frequently during the course of the disease in patients with glioma and challenge the definition of RANO criteria progression, as they do not fulfil the criteria for RANO progression.

- Speckled contrast-enhancing lesions are found more frequently in astrocytoma WHO grade II and III, in oligodendroglial tumors, and in IDH mutant glioma. Although they are usually relatively benign and may stay stable or dissolve, they are continually a source of clinical and patient concern.
- Clinical practice emphasizes cautious definitions of progression and regular clinical and MRI follow-up rather than premature initiation of new antitumor therapies until

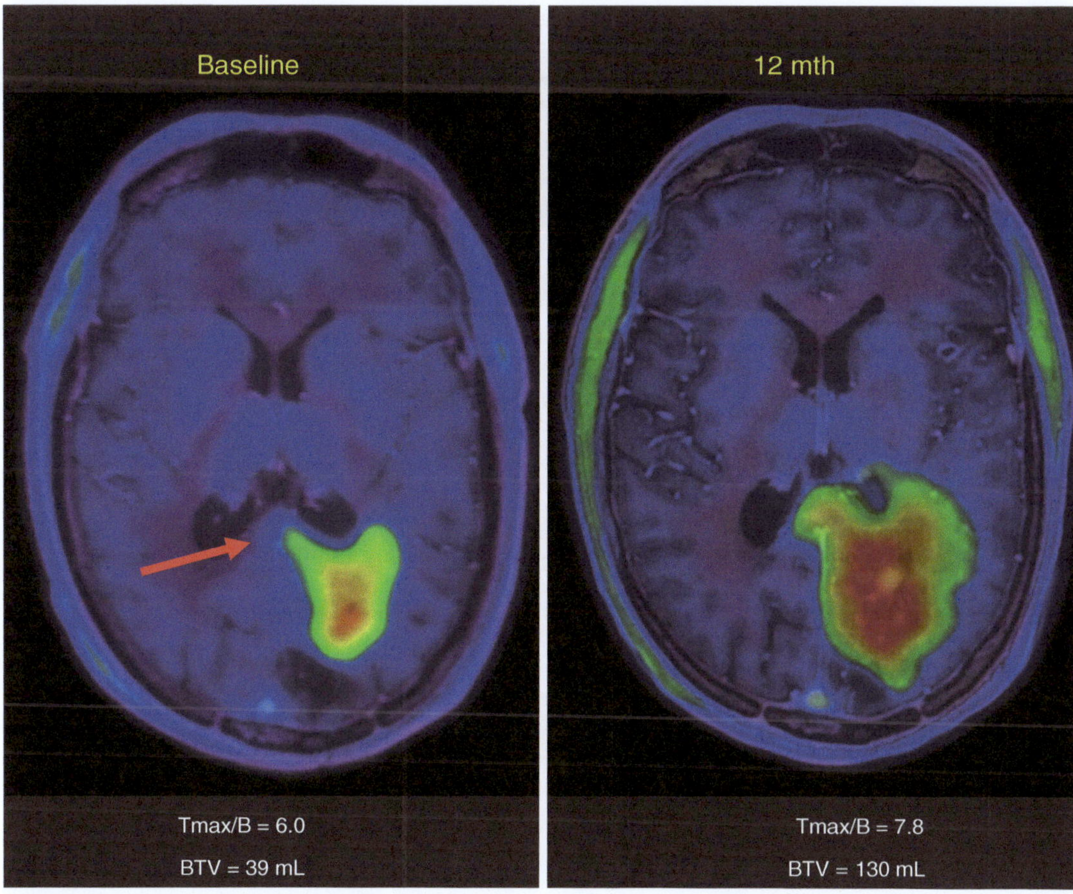


**Fig. 3** PET scans using [$^{18}$F]FET fused to T1 postcontrast MRI at the same positions and conditions as in Fig. 1. At baseline marked active tumor is identified in the left parietooccipital region, demonstrating viable tumor tissue despite stable conditions on MRI. Activity in the splenium (red arrow) could not be identified despite FLAIR signal changes. Progression and treatment failure during chemotherapy at 12 months are measured by maximal tumor to background ratio (Tmax/B) and biological tumor volume (BTV)

progression is confirmed preferably with measurable contrast enhancement (>10 × 10 mm).

- MRI evaluation of glioma that progress *without* significant contrast enhancement rely on T2 FLAIR hyperintensity signal changes, where tumor measures are less certain.
- T2 FLAIR signal hyperintensity may arise because of tumor infiltration, but unspecific increases in FLAIR signal may be secondary to surgery, radiation, or chemotherapy, representing edema, gliosis, demyelination, or ischemia.
- Amino acid PET tracers, such as O-(2-[$^{18}$F] fluoroethyl)-L-tyrosine ([$^{18}$F]FET), are transported into glioma by the L-amino transporter (LAT) independent of a blood–brain barrier disruption and is particularly useful in non-contrast-enhancing tumors.

## Imaging Findings

- [$^{18}$F]FET PET can show increased activity in MRI with or without concomitant contrast, non-contrast-enhancing signal changes.
- Oligodendroglioma is usually very active.
- Non-contrast-enhancing signal changes may be unspecific without increased [$^{18}$F]FET uptake (Fig. 3).

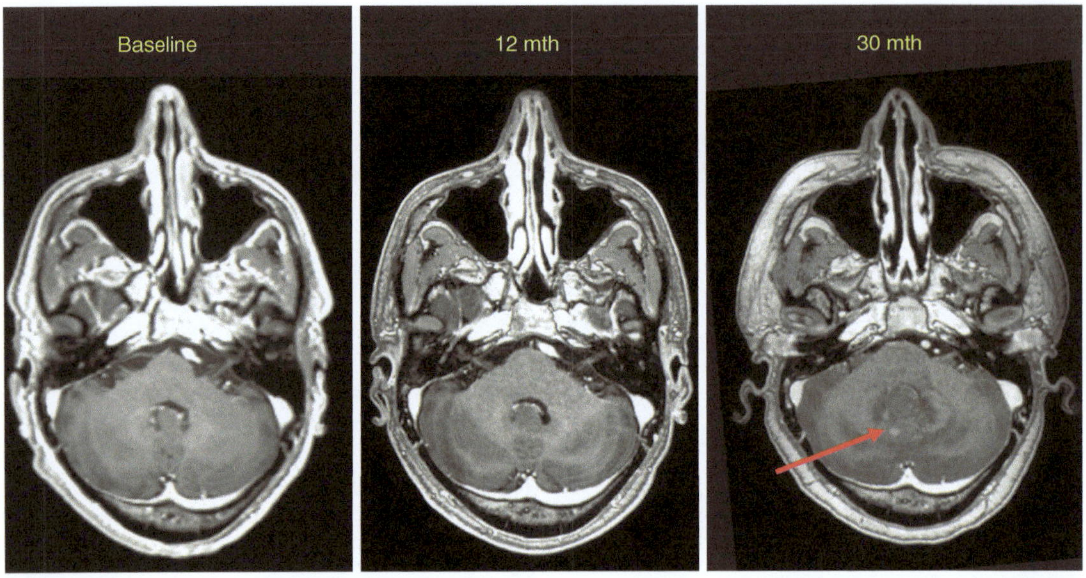


**Fig. 4** T1 postcontrast MRI at the level of the vermis showing no contrast-enhancing tumor tissue before MRI follow-up at 30 months (red arrow)

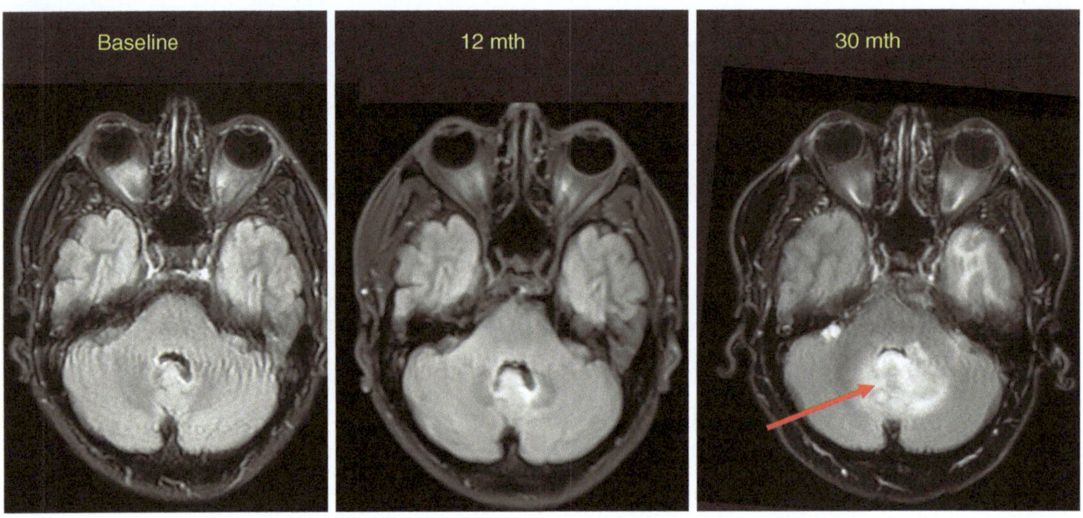


**Fig. 5** T2 FLAIR MRI at the same positions as in Fig. 4 showing uncertain signal changes in the vermis at 12 months that become manifest on later MRI follow-ups (red arrow)

## Clinical Management

- Amino acid PET disease is an important decision tool in management of patients with uncertain MRI.
- [$^{18}$F]FET PET can aid in the identification of metabolically active tumor tissue and treatment failure and can provide evidence of more extensive spread. Distant metastases will usually exclude re-resection.
- The documentation of active tumor tissue with [$^{18}$F]FET PET scan supported the initiation in this patient of temozolomide and later antiangiogenic therapy.

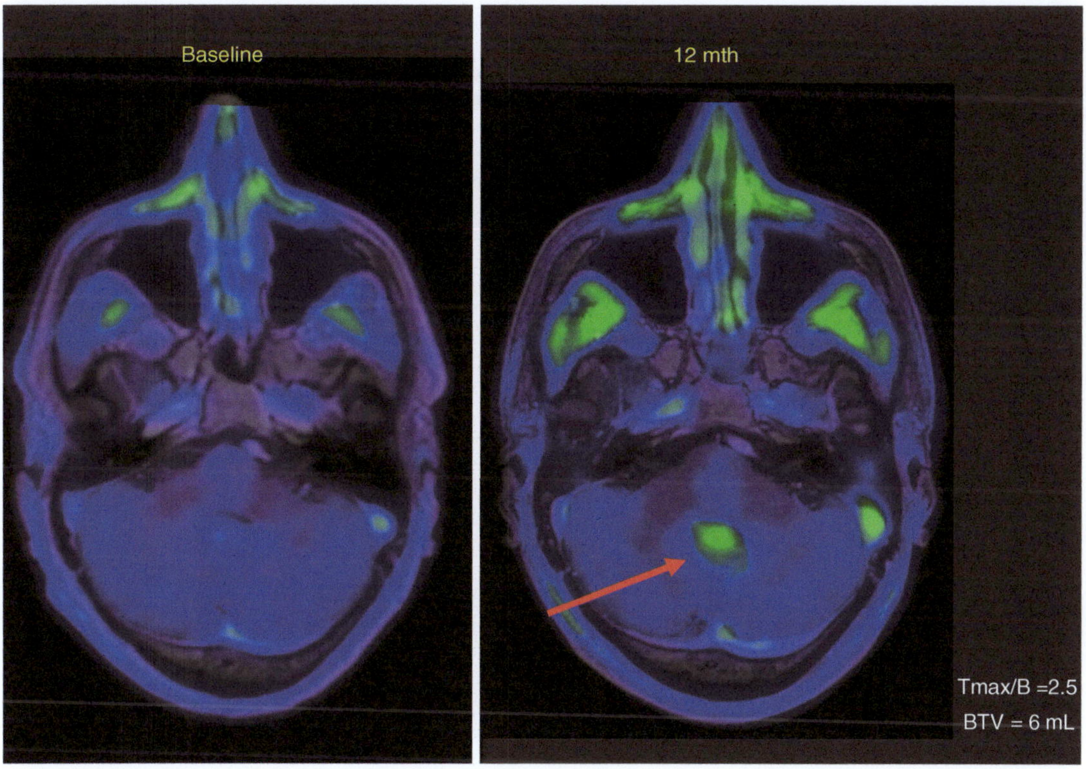


**Fig. 6** [18F]FET PET fused to T1 postcontrast MRI at the same positions as in Fig. 4. A new lesion with moderate focal increase in the vermis adjacent to the 4th ventricle, indicating distant malignant spread (red arrow)

**Take-Home Message**

- Amino acid PET imaging may improve assessment of disease burden and treatment response and planning in select glioma patients, and allow for identification of distant spread that is not readily identified on conventional MRI.

## Further Reading

Albert NL, Weller M, Suchorska B, et al. Response assessment in neuro-oncology working group and European Association for Neuro-Oncology recommendations for the clinical use of PET imaging in gliomas. Neuro-Oncology. 2016;18(9):1199–208.

Berberich A, Hielscher T, Kickingereder P, et al. Nonmeasurable speckled contrast-enhancing lesions appearing during course of disease are associated with IDH mutation in high-grade astrocytoma patients. Int J Radiat Oncol Biol Phys. 2018;102(5):1472–80.

Galldiks N, Law I, Pope WB, Arbizu J, Langen KJ. The use of amino acid PET and conventional MRI for monitoring of brain tumor therapy. Neuroimage Clin. 2017;13:386–94.

Law I, Albert NL, Arbizu J, et al. Joint EANM/EANO/RANO practice guidelines/SNMMI procedure standards for imaging of gliomas using PET with radiolabelled amino acids and [18F]FDG: version 1.0. Eur J Nucl Med Mol Imaging. 2019;46:540–57.

# Case 25: Primary Diagnosis of an Isocitrate Dehydrogenase (IDH) Wild-Type Glioma

Nathalie L. Albert, Bogdana Suchorska, Adrien Holzgreve, and Marcus Unterrainer

A 73-year-old male patient presented with a generalized tonic-clonic seizure at the emergency department. The patient was agitated, poorly oriented, and had a Glasgow Coma Scale (GCS) score of 7. He showed no targeted defense against pain stimuli, presented with a generalized increase in tonicity and undirected movements of all four extremities. The pupils were narrow and isochoric. A cranial CT was performed, which revealed an intra-axial mass in the left parietal lobe with a size of approximately 2.5 × 2.0 cm, surrounding perifocal, vasogenic edema as well as partly pin-shaped calcifications (see Fig. 1a). A moderate local volume effect with compression on the left posterior horn of the lateral ventricle was seen, no relevant midline shift. No intracranial bleeding was found.

As the laboratory examinations revealed a massive increase in creatine kinase and myoglobin and a Crush syndrome-related kidney failure was diagnosed due to seizure-related rhabdomyolysis, the patient was hospitalized and observed in the intensive care unit. The contrast-enhanced MRI could not be performed until improvement of his condition and normalization of the kidney function 12 days later.

The MRI showed a hypo-intense mass on the T1w images with two circumscribed structures with very subtle contrast enhancement (see Fig. 1b). In combination with the calcifications found on the CT scan, an oligodendroglioma was suspected.

An additional amino acid PET scan using O-(2-$^{18}$F-fluoroethyl)-L-tyrosine ([$^{18}$F]FET) was performed subsequently, revealing a bifocal and intense [$^{18}$F]FET enhancement in the left parietal lobe, which correlated with the subtle bifocal contrast enhancement found in the T1w MRI sequence (see Fig. 1d). The maximal tumor-to-background ratio was 3.5, the dynamic evaluation showed a very early peak at 7 min followed by clearly decreasing curves (see Fig. 1e).

After the completion of noninvasive diagnostics, a stereotactic biopsy was performed to assess tissue samples for final histological diagnosis; a surgical resection was not possible due to the patient's poor clinical condition. The neuropathological analysis revealed an anaplastic astrocytoma (WHO grade III). No 1p/19q codeletion could be found in the genetic analyses, therefore excluding an oligodendroglioma.

N. L. Albert (✉) · A. Holzgreve
Department of Nuclear Medicine, University Hospital, LMU Munich, Munich, Germany
e-mail: nathalie.albert@med.uni-muenchen.de; Adrien.holzgreve@med.uni-muenchen.de

B. Suchorska
Department of Neurosurgery, University Hospital, LMU Munich, Munich, Germany
e-mail: bogdana.suchorska@med.uni-muenchen.de; bogdana.suchorska@sana.de

M. Unterrainer
Department of Nuclear Medicine, University Hospital, LMU Munich, Munich, Germany

Department of Radiology, University Hospital, LMU Munich, Munich, Germany
e-mail: Marcus.unterrainer@med.uni-muenchen.de



A. Varrone et al. (eds.), *Clinical Nuclear Medicine in Neurology*,
https://doi.org/10.1007/978-3-030-83598-9_25

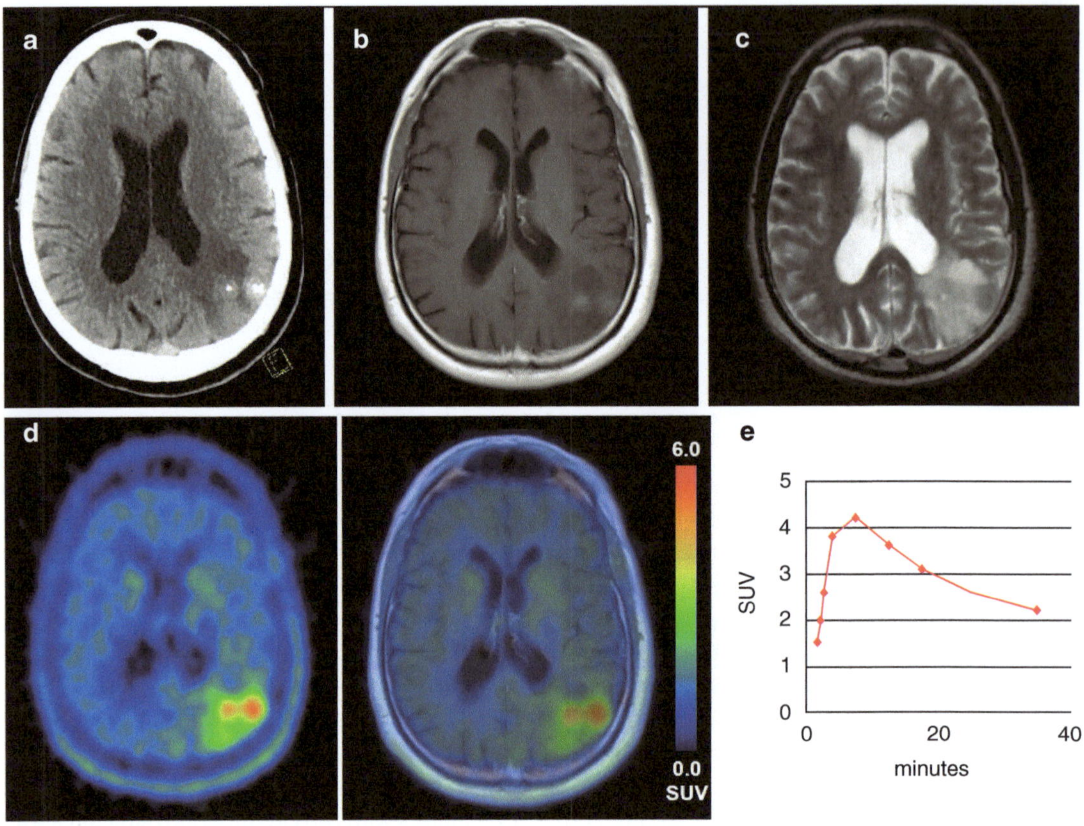


**Fig. 1** (**a**) CT scan with calcifications of the mass in the left parietal lobe, (**b**) contrast-enhanced T1-weighted MRI showing subtle contrast enhancement, (**c**) T2-weighted MRI with perifocal edema, (**d**) static $[^{18}F]$FET PET images (on the right side fused with the MRI) showing a bifocal intense amino acid uptake, (**e**) dynamic analysis of the tumoral tracer uptake showing decreasing time–activity curves after an early peak uptake

Furthermore, no mutation of the isocitrate dehydrogenase (IDH) 1/2 was found. The integrated diagnosis according to the 2016 updated WHO classification was an *IDH* wild-type glioma WHO grade III which is known to have a comparably poor prognosis as glioblastoma [1], which led to the treatment decision of a combined radiochemotherapy following patient's clinical improvement.

Although the newly diagnosed intracranial mass did not present with the typical findings for a glioblastoma (i.e., contrast enhancement on MRI with central necrosis), and even mimicked an oligodendroglial tumor on CT (calcifications), the latter one being associated with a relatively good prognosis, the PET findings gave a hint toward the correct diagnosis. In the past decade, amino acid PET using $[^{18}F]$FET, L-methyl-$^{11}$C-methionine ($[^{11}C]$MET), or $[^{18}F]$ fluoro-dihydroxyphenylalanine ($[^{18}F]$DOPA) has been increasingly used for the assessment of glioma patients. Besides its use for treatment planning, treatment evaluation and the differentiation between tumor recurrence and treatment-induced changes, it has been recommended for the assessment of newly diagnosed, glioma-suspicious lesions [2]. While older studies have evaluated the performance of amino acid PET for tumor grading [3–7], more recent studies are focusing on the prediction of the *IDH* mutation status [8–11]. In this context, particularly the evaluation of uptake *dynamics* was reported to enable a differentiation between *IDH* mutant and *IDH* wild-type gliomas [8, 11], while static parameters alone are not sufficient for the prediction.

Coming back to the reported case with suspected oligodendroglioma (i.e., *IDH* mutant tumor with 1p/19q codeletion), the high tracer uptake intensity on [$^{18}$F]FET PET would in general also have been compatible with an oligodendroglial tumor; however, the very short time-to-peak of 7 min controverts the diagnosis of an *IDH* mutant tumor [8]. Decreasing curves after a short time-to-peak are usually associated with a poor prognosis [12] and are highly suggestive for an *IDH* wild-type glioma, even if only subtle contrast enhancement can be found on MRI [8].

Taken together, dynamic [$^{18}$F]FET PET with analysis of the tracer kinetics can be of great help to assess the entity of an unclear glioma-suspicious lesion. Importantly, [$^{18}$F]FET PET can even be applied in patients with impaired kidney function, who would not be suitable for contrast-enhanced MRI.

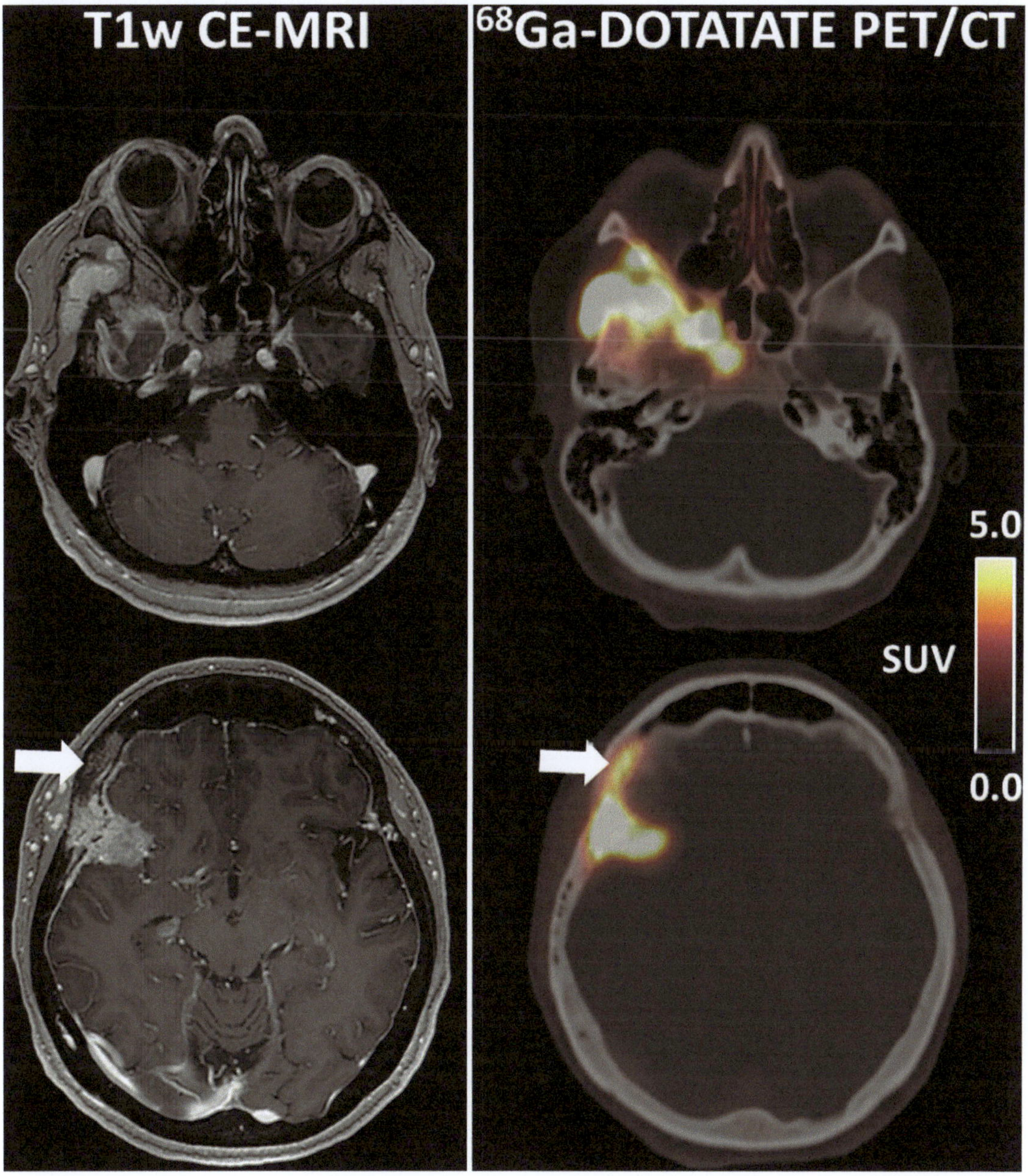

## References


1. Louis DN, Perry A, Reifenberger G, von Deimling A, Figarella-Branger D, Cavenee WK, et al. The 2016 World Health Organization Classification of Tumors of the Central Nervous System: a summary. Acta Neuropathol. 2016;131(6):803–20.
2. Albert NL, Weller M, Suchorska B, Galldiks N, Soffietti R, Kim MM, et al. Response Assessment in Neuro-Oncology working group and European Association for Neuro-Oncology recommendations for the clinical use of PET imaging in gliomas. Neuro-Oncology. 2016;18(9):1199–208.
3. Dunet V, Pomoni A, Hottinger A, Nicod-Lalonde M, Prior JO. Performance of 18F-FET versus 18F-FDG-PET for the diagnosis and grading of brain tumors: systematic review and meta-analysis. Neuro-Oncology. 2015;18(3):426–34.
4. Albert NL, Winkelmann I, Suchorska B, Wenter V, Schmid-Tannwald C, Mille E, et al. Early static (18) F-FET-PET scans have a higher accuracy for glioma grading than the standard 20-40 min scans. Eur J Nucl Med Mol Imaging. 2016;43(6):1105–14.
5. Calcagni ML, Galli G, Giordano A, Taralli S, Anile C, Niesen A, et al. Dynamic O-(2-[18F]fluoroethyl)-L-tyrosine (F-18 FET) PET for glioma grading: assessment of individual probability of malignancy. Clin Nucl Med. 2011;36(10):841–7.
6. Jansen NL, Graute V, Armbruster L, Suchorska B, Lutz J, Eigenbrod S, et al. MRI-suspected low-grade glioma: is there a need to perform dynamic FET PET? Eur J Nucl Med Mol Imaging. 2012;39(6):1021–9.
7. Lohmann P, Herzog H, Rota Kops E, Stoffels G, Judov N, Filss C, et al. Dual-time-point O-(2-[F] fluoroethyl)-L-tyrosine PET for grading of cerebral gliomas. Eur Radiol. 2015;25(10):3017–24.
8. Vettermann F, Suchorska B, Unterrainer M, Nelwan D, Forbrig R, Ruf V, et al. Non-invasive prediction of IDH-wildtype genotype in gliomas using dynamic (18)F-FET PET. Eur J Nucl Med Mol Imaging. 2019;46(12):2581.
9. Bumes E, Wirtz FP, Fellner C, Grosse J, Hellwig D, Oefner PJ, et al. Non-invasive prediction of IDH mutation in patients with glioma WHO II/III/IV Based on F-18-FET PET-guided in vivo (1)H-magnetic resonance spectroscopy and machine learning. Cancer. 2020;12:11.
10. Zaragori T, Guedj E, Verger A. Is IDH mutation status associated with (18)F-FDopa PET uptake? Ann Nucl Med. 2020;34(3):228–9.
11. Ginet M, Zaragori T, Marie PY, Roch V, Gauchotte G, Rech F, et al. Integration of dynamic parameters in the analysis of (18)F-FDopa PET imaging improves the prediction of molecular features of gliomas. Eur J Nucl Med Mol Imaging. 2020;47(6):1381–90.
12. Suchorska B, Giese A, Biczok A, Unterrainer M, Weller M, Drexler M, et al. Identification of time-to-peak on dynamic 18F-FET-PET as a prognostic marker specifically in IDH1/2 mutant diffuse astrocytoma. Neuro-Oncology. 2017;20(2):279–88.

# Case 26: Postoperative Meningioma

Ian Law and Asma Bashir

## Patient

A 54-year-old woman with atypical meningioma (WHO II) in the left frontal lobe. Prior to diagnosis, the patient suffered from almost constant frontal headaches, nausea, excessive sleepiness, and slight weakness of the right arm. Resection was performed. MRI 3 months postoperative showed slight contrast enhancement without certain tumor remnants.

## Epidemiology

Meningiomas are the most common primary intracranial tumors (37%) with an average annual age-adjusted incidence rate of (8 per 100,000 population).

## Pathology

- Neurofibromatose type II is a risk factor for meningioma.
- Most meningiomas are classified as WHO grade I (80%), with fewer classified as WHO grade II (18%) or grade III lesions (2%) on the basis of local invasiveness and cellular features of atypia.
- Meningioma has a tendency to recur dependent on WHO grade, remnant tumor tissue, molecular features (TERT mutation), and methylation profile.
- Meningioma may invade vasculature, bone and muscle, and incase vasculature and cranial nerves.
- The majority of meningiomas show expression of somatostatin receptor 2 (SSRT2).

## Background

- Radiolabeled somatostatin receptor analogues bind strongly to SSRT2 in meningiomas.
- Several PET tracers are implemented in clinical use, e.g., DOTA-D-Phe$^{1}$-Tyr$^{3}$-octreotide labeled with Gallium-68 ([$^{68}$Ga]Ga-DOTA-TOC).

## Imaging Findings

- The primary presentation of meningiomas is usually well-delineated extra-axial solitary round tumors found on MRI or CT with rela-

I. Law (✉)
Department of Clinical Physiology, Nuclear Medicine and PET, University of Copenhagen, Copenhagen, Denmark
e-mail: ian.law@regionh.dk

A. Bashir
Department of Neurosurgery, Rigshospitalet, University of Copenhagen, Copenhagen, Denmark



A. Varrone et al. (eds.), *Clinical Nuclear Medicine in Neurology*,
https://doi.org/10.1007/978-3-030-83598-9_26

tionship to the dura mater displacing the cortex and with strong enhancement after contrast injection (Fig. 1).

- Focal or irregular high contrast [$^{68}$Ga]Ga-DOTA-TOC uptake (Fig. 2)
  - Associated to overt contrast-enhancing tumor, e.g., in the orbit.
- Or evading identification on MRI.
  - Adjacent to the resection cavity in unspecific contrast enhancing areas on MRI.
  - In bone seen as osteosclerotic or osteolytic changes on CT.
  - In muscle of mastication/face.
  - Infiltrating into cranial openings in the scull base.
  - Intravascularly adjacent or in sinuses and jugular veins.

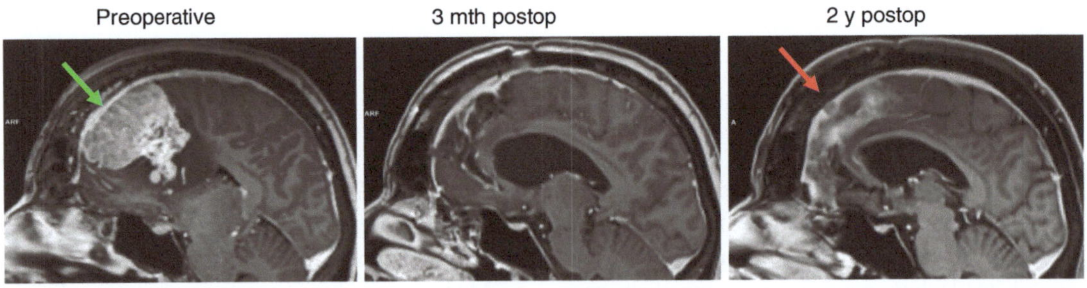


**Fig. 1** Sagittal T1 MRI postcontrast images of large contrast-enhancing meningioma in the left frontal lobe with close association to the sagittal sinus (green arrow) showing atypical WHO grade II on pathology. MRI follow-ups 3 months and 2 years post resection are reported without certain tumor remnant or recurrence

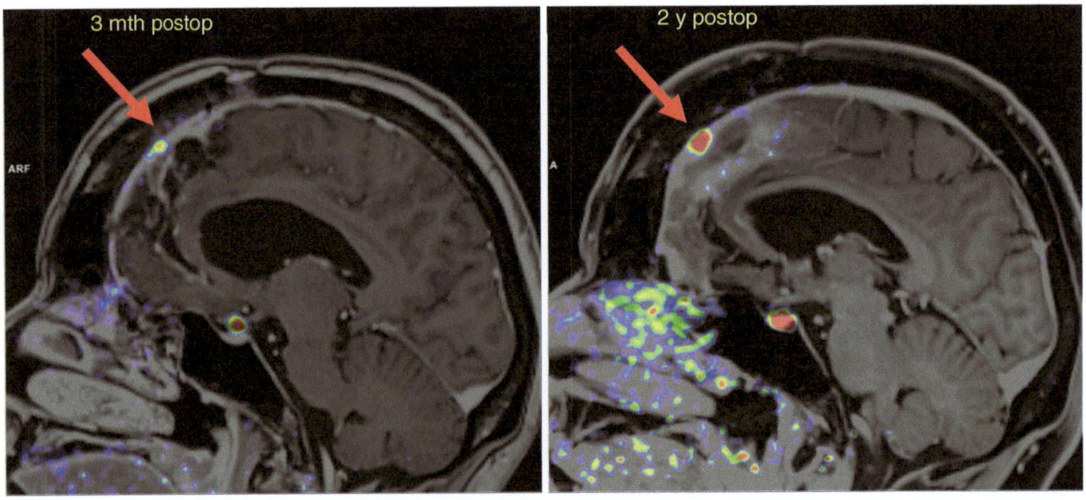


**Fig. 2** Sagittal slices as in Fig. 1 showing PET scans using [$^{68}$Ga]Ga-DOTA-TOC fused to T1 postcontrast MRI. At 3 months follow-up, a small focal remnant is found close to the sagittal sinus (0.2 mL, red arrow) in unspecific contrast enhancement on MRI. Repeated PET scanning after 2 years in order to follow-up the initial suspected remnant showed growth (0.7 mL) and was found retrospectively to coincide with a gray nodular tumor intravascularly in the sagittal sinus confirming the initial finding. The patient was asymptomatic

## Clinical Management

- Gross total resection of WHO grade I meningiomas in favorable locations can be curative.
- Residual or remnant tumor tissue can be followed by MRI for evidence of further progression or treated up-front with surgery or radiation therapy. There is no established recommendation for chemotherapy.

**Take-Home Message**

[$^{68}$Ga]Ga-DOTA-TOC PET imaging is particularly useful in detecting active meningioma remnants at locations and conditions difficult for MRI, e.g., in posttreatment damage, at the scull base, in bone, vascular structures, skin, and muscle. [$^{68}$Ga]Ga-DOTA-TOC PET can aid management by early tumor detection, improved tumor delineation for radiation therapy and surgical resection, and separation of recurrent tumor from radiation damage.

## Further Reading

Bashir A, Larsen VA, Ziebell M, Fugleholm K, Law I. Improved Detection of Postoperative Residual Meningioma with [68Ga]Ga-DOTA-TOC PET Imaging Using a High-resolution Research Tomograph PET Scanner. Clin Cancer Res. 2021;27:2216–25.

Galldiks N, Albert NL, Sommerauer M, et al. PET imaging in patients with meningioma – report of the RANO/PET Group. Neuro Oncol. 2017;19(12):1576–87.

Ueberschaer M, Vettermann FJ, Forbrig R, et al. Simpson grade revisited - intraoperative estimation of the extent of resection in meningiomas versus postoperative somatostatin receptor positron emission tomography/computed tomography and magnetic resonance imaging. Neurosurgery. 2020;88(1):140–6.

# Case 27: Meningioma with Difficult Delineation on MRI

Adrien Holzgreve, Marcus Unterrainer, Bogdana Suchorska, and Nathalie L. Albert

A 57-year-old female patient presented with progressive swelling of the right temple. A previously performed MRI scan exhibited a large tumor at the right sphenoid wing with extensive infiltration of surrounding osseous structures and of the right temporal muscle. The patient was fully oriented, and there were no neurological deficits or functional impairment of cranial nerves. Further neurological examination was unremarkable. Ophthalmologic evaluation revealed right eye proptosis without visual impairment or diplopia.

For treatment planning, a high-resolution contrast-enhanced MRI was performed (see left row in the figure). MRI exhibited a large, homogenously contrast-enhancing lesion predominantly located in the right temporal lobe with transosseous growth and infiltration of the right temporal muscle. The lateral wall of the orbital cavity was thickened and showed contrast enhancement. The greater wing of the right sphenoid bone was distended. Additional lesions suspicious for a tumor were not detected.

For further evaluation of tumor delineation and extent of bone involvement, a combined PET/CT scan with gallium-68 ($^{68}$Ga)-DOTA-D-Phe1-Tyr3-octreotate ([$^{68}$Ga]DOTATATE) PET and contrast-enhanced CT was performed (see right row in the figure). Here, a high [$^{68}$Ga]DOTATATE uptake of the lesion was noted (SUVmax 23.7), indicating a strong somatostatin receptor (SSTR) expression, which is highly suggestive of a meningioma. In the superior direction, the tumor extended up to the Sylvian fissure. In the inferior direction, the mass showed partial destruction of the sphenoid bone and infiltrative growth into the infratemporal fossa, the pterygopalatine fossa, and the temporal muscle. In the medial direction, the lesion nearly reached the pituitary gland. In the anterior direction, an infiltration of the lateral posterior portion of the bony orbital process was noted. The craniocaudal extension of the mass was 8.1 cm; the extension in axial plane was 4.4 × 4.1 cm.

A PET/CT-navigated microsurgical tumor resection including partial resection of the involved bony structures and orbital decompression was performed. There was no postoperative neurological deficit. Histopathology revealed a WHO grade I transitional meningioma. Follow-up

A. Holzgreve · N. L. Albert (✉)
Department of Nuclear Medicine, University Hospital, LMU Munich, Munich, Germany
e-mail: Adrien.Holzgreve@med.uni-muenchen.de; Nathalie.Albert@med.uni-muenchen.de

M. Unterrainer
Department of Nuclear Medicine, University Hospital, LMU Munich, Munich, Germany

Department of Radiology, University Hospital, LMU Munich, Munich, Germany
e-mail: Marcus.Unterrainer@med.uni-muenchen.de

B. Suchorska
Department of Neurosurgery, University Hospital, LMU Munich, Munich, Germany
e-mail: bogdana.suchorska@med.uni-muenchen.de



A. Varrone et al. (eds.), *Clinical Nuclear Medicine in Neurology*,
https://doi.org/10.1007/978-3-030-83598-9_27

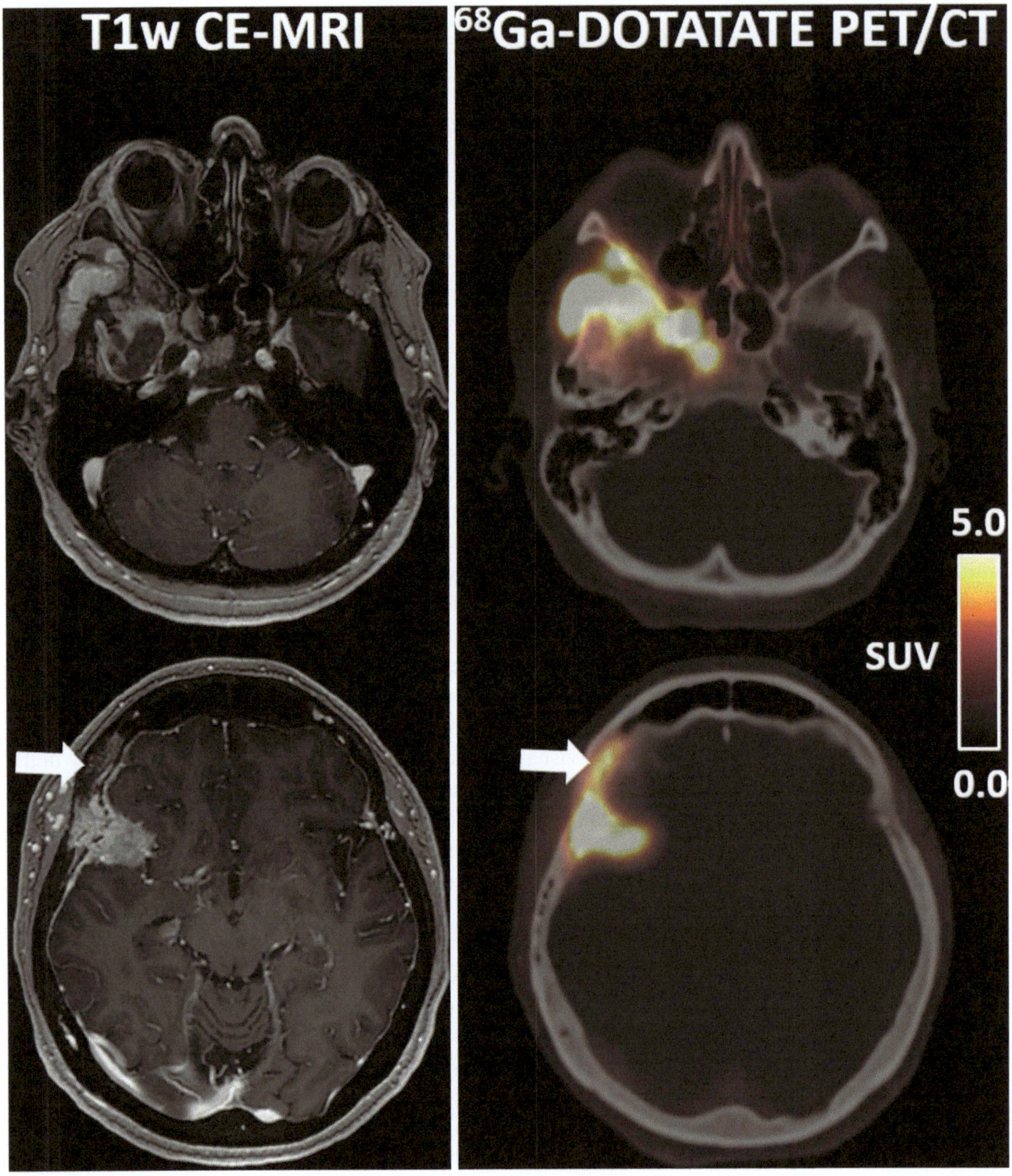


MRI examinations 3 months as well as 15 months later revealed no residual or recurrent tumor.

In clinical routine, the delineation of skull base meningiomas can be challenging as the imaging gold standard MRI alone is limited in depicting the extent of osseous infiltration of the tumor. However, local therapies such as surgical resection and radiotherapy, which are the mainstay of meningioma treatment, require accurate prior tumor delineation [1]. Therefore, additional advanced methods are warranted for meningioma imaging. Especially PET imaging with SSTR-targeted tracers such as [$^{68}$Ga]DOTATATE, [$^{68}$Ga]DOTA-Tyr3-octreotide ([$^{68}$Ga]DOTATOC), and [$^{68}$Ga]DOTA-1-Nal3-

octreotide ([$^{68}$Ga]DOTANOC) has proven to be beneficial for meningioma evaluation [2–4]. Although mainly restricted to centers with a $^{68}$Ge/$^{68}$Ga generator, SSTR-targeted PET has widely been accepted as a valuable complementary diagnostic tool in the clinical management of meningioma patients owing to its role in precise delineation of meningioma as illustrated in the current case, in contribution to treatment stratification, as well as to its ability in differentiating residual or recurrent tumor from postsurgical or radiation treatment-related changes [5, 6]. For instance, in the current case, the use of preoperative PET/CT imaging for treatment planning allowed for a more extensive tumor resection as the SSTR-targeted PET component either confirmed unclear tumor margins or even depicted vital tumor tissue beyond the visible tumor extent in gold standard MRI (e. g., see white arrows). Furthermore, especially taking the patient's age into account, lesions of a different histopathological origin such as metastasis or sarcoidosis, could be excluded.

The current applications of PET imaging in meningioma patients are valuable for the clinical management and will further profit from validation in studies with larger patient cohorts. Additional perspectives for nuclear medicine in meningioma imaging include the development and implementation of more widely available $^{18}$F-labeled SSR-targeted tracers, the noninvasive extraction of specific biological and prognostic information as well as the evaluation of theranostic treatment concepts [7–9].

## References

1. Goldbrunner R, Minniti G, Preusser M, Jenkinson MD, Sallabanda K, Houdart E, et al. EANO guidelines for the diagnosis and treatment of meningiomas. Lancet Oncol. 2016;17(9):e383–91.
2. Galldiks N, Albert NL, Sommerauer M, Grosu AL, Ganswindt U, Law I, et al. PET imaging in patients with meningioma-report of the RANO/PET Group. Neuro-Oncology. 2017;19(12):1576–87.
3. Nowosielski M, Galldiks N, Iglseder S, Kickingereder P, von Deimling A, Bendszus M, et al. Diagnostic challenges in meningioma. Neuro-Oncology. 2017;19(12):1588–98.
4. Kunz WG, Jungblut LM, Kazmierczak PM, Vettermann FJ, Bollenbacher A, Tonn JC, et al. Improved detection of transosseous meningiomas using (68)Ga-DOTATATE PET/CT compared with contrast-enhanced MRI. J Nucl Med. 2017;58(10):1580–7.
5. Huang RY, Bi WL, Griffith B, Kaufmann TJ, la Fougère C, Schmidt NO, et al. Imaging and diagnostic advances for intracranial meningiomas. Neuro-Oncology. 2019;21(Suppl 1):44–61.
6. Brastianos PK, Galanis E, Butowski N, Chan JW, Dunn IF, Goldbrunner R, et al. Advances in multidisciplinary therapy for meningiomas. Neuro-Oncology. 2019;21(Suppl 1):18–31.
7. Bashir A, Vestergaard MB, Marner L, Larsen VA, Ziebell M, Fugleholm K, et al. PET imaging of meningioma with 18F-FLT: a predictor of tumour progression. Brain. 2020;143(11):3308–17.
8. Lindner S, Wängler C, Bailey JJ, Jurkschat K, Bartenstein P, Wängler B, et al. Radiosynthesis of [(18)F]SiFAlin-TATE for clinical neuroendocrine tumor positron emission tomography. Nat Protoc. 2020;15(12):3827–43.
9. Seystahl K, Stoecklein V, Schüller U, Rushing E, Nicolas G, Schäfer N, et al. Somatostatin receptor-targeted radionuclide therapy for progressive meningioma: benefit linked to 68Ga-DOTATATE/-TOC uptake. Neuro-Oncology. 2016;18(11):1538–47.

# Case 28: Optic Nerve Sheath Meningioma (ONSM)

Tatiana Horowitz, Betty Salgues, and Eric Guedj

## Case Summary

A 17-year-old woman was referred for the management of a progressive right visual loss. She had a medical history of headache. Ophthalmological examination revealed a major right papilledema with a blind spot enlargement and a right exophthalmos. The rest of the clinical examination was normal. MRI showed a right intra-orbital tumor, isointense on T1-weighted images, with peripheral enhancement, and no intracranial extension. An optic nerve sheath meningioma (ONSM) was suspected and a [$^{68}$Ga] DOTATOC PET-CT contributed to the diagnosis by showing overexpression of SSRT2 of the lesion. She recovered visual acuity after fractioned stereotactic radiotherapy treatment, without complication.

A 17-year-old woman with unilateral loss of vision acuity revealing an ONSM (Figs. 1 and 2)

## Epidemiology

- Rare meningioma location, accounts for 1–2% of meningioma.
- Also rare etiology of orbital tumors (2%).

T. Horowitz · B. Salgues · E. Guedj (✉)
Nuclear Medicine Department, Aix Marseille Univ, APHM, CNRS, Centrale Marseille, Institut Fresnel, Timone Hospital, CERIMED, Marseille, France
e-mail: eric.guedj@univ-amu.fr

## Pathology

- Benign tumor originated from arachnoids' cells of optic nerve sheath.

## Clinical Features

- Progressive loss of vision acuity, exophthalmos.
- Optic nerve edema and optic pallor.
- Exophthalmos can be missing, leading to frequent misdiagnose.

## Clinical Management

- Surgical resection is often impossible due to location.
- Stereotactic radiotherapy can be proposed with risks of radiation-induced retinopathy or optic neuropathy.
- Somatostatin receptor-targeted radiopeptide therapy is under study for SSTR2-positive meningioma.

## Imaging Findings

- MRI shows isointense T1 and T2 tumor with outer enhancing of the ONSM and inner non-enhancing optic nerve corresponding to the "tram-track" sign.



A. Varrone et al. (eds.), *Clinical Nuclear Medicine in Neurology*,
https://doi.org/10.1007/978-3-030-83598-9_28

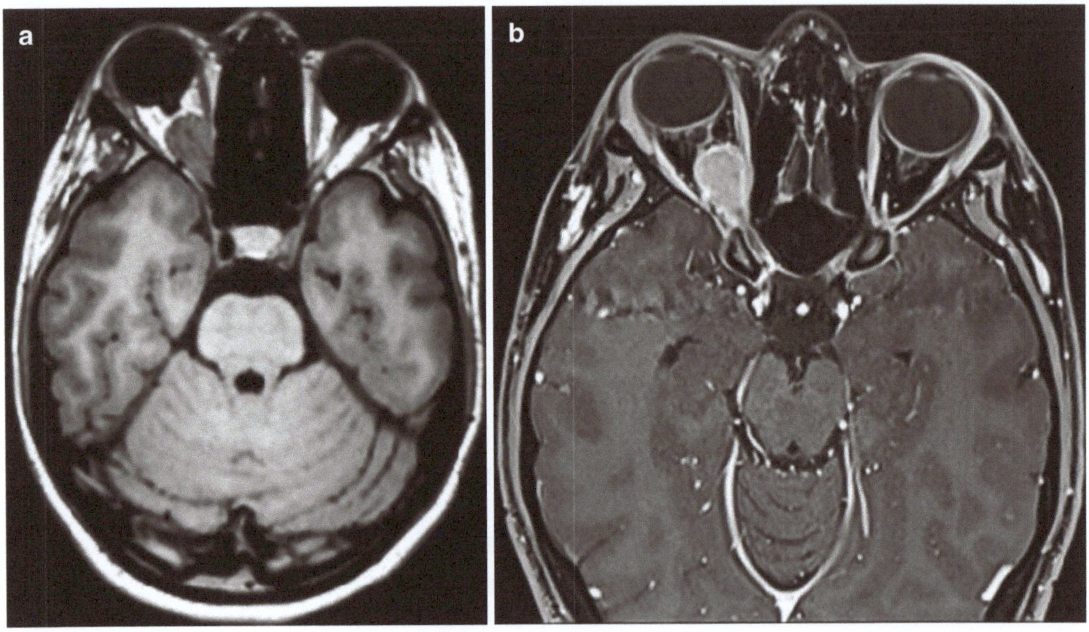


**Fig. 1** Axial MRI T1-weighted slices showing a right intra-orbital tumor (**a**) with peripheral enhancement after gadolinium injection (**b**)

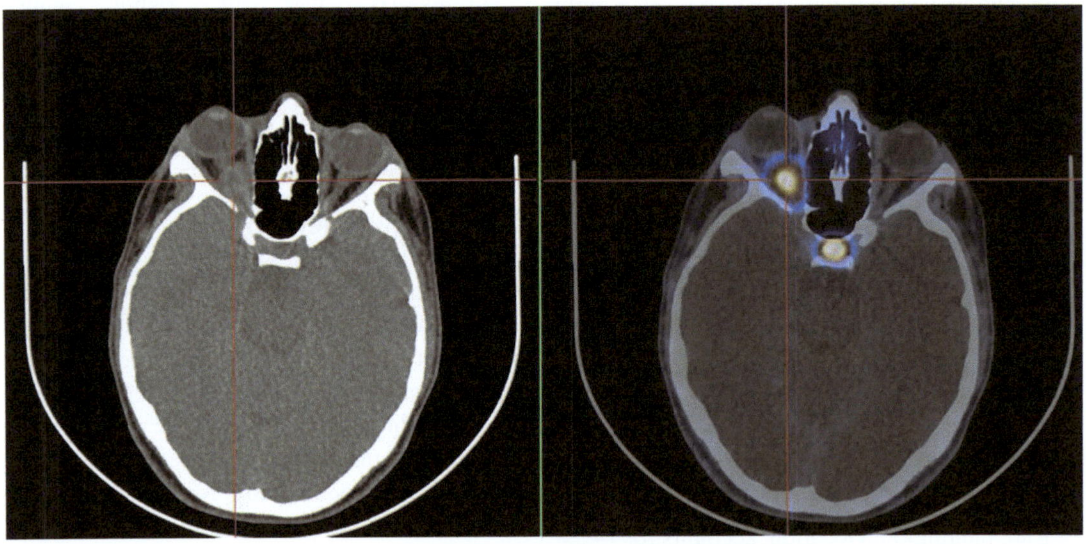

**Fig. 2** Axial [68Ga]DOTATOC PET-CT fused and CT slices showing overexpression of somatostatin receptor subtype 2 (SSRT2) of the right intra-orbital mass, suggestive of a meningioma. No remote lesion was identified

- Differential diagnosis with optical nerve glioma or lymphoma can be difficult on MRI.
- Since meningiomas generally express SST2 receptors, [68Ga]DOTATOC PET-CT shows intense tracer uptake.

**Take-Home Message**
- [68Ga]DOTATOC PET-CT can be useful for the diagnosis of suspected meningioma, and can differentiate optic nerve glioma and lymphoma from ONSM.

## Further Reading

Afshar-Oromieh A, Giesel FL, Linhart HG, Haberkorn U, Haufe S, Combs SE, Podlesek D, Eisenhut M, Kratochwil C. Detection of cranial meningiomas: comparison of $^{68}$Ga-DOTATOC PET/CT and contrast-enhanced MRI. Eur J Nucl Med Mol Imaging. 2012;39(9):1409–15.

Kahraman-Koytak P, Bruce BB, Peragallo JH, Newman NJ, Biousse V. Diagnostic errors in initial misdiagnosis of optic nerve sheath meningiomas. JAMA Neurol. 2019;76(3):326–32.

# Case 29: Primary Brain Lymphoma

Javier Arbizu and Juan Fernando Bastidas

## Case Summary

A 64-year-old immunocompetent man with a 3-day history of bradypsychia and behavioral disorder. Patient progressively presented cephalea, gait disturbance, alexia, and agraphia. The clinical examination showed right body lateropulsion, dysmetria in the right limbs and diplopia.

## Images/Findings

A brain CT performed at the emergency room showed a brain tumor in the left mesencephalon. Brain magnetic resonance imaging (MRI) on the T1 sequences with gadolinium demonstrated a focal area of contrast enhancement without a clear area of necrosis with a size of 16 × 18 mm in (Fig. 1). The T2 Flair shows a hypointense lesion (suggestive of hypercellularity) surrounded by an area of hyperintensity (suggestive of edema and/or infiltrative component) with a size of 30 × 23 mm (Fig. 2). The perfusion study shows increased values, around five times the value of the contralateral with matter. The images were suspicious of a high-grade glioma vs. cerebral lymphoma in the left mesencephalon that extends to basal ganglia. A positron emission tomography (PET/CT) study was proposed in order to characterize the lesion as well as to stage a possible systemic disease.

The whole-body PET/CT scan with [$^{18}$F]fluorodeoxyglucose (FDG-PET) showed a markedly increased uptake of the radiotracer on the brain lesion located on the left mesencephalon extending from the cerebral peduncle toward the thalamus and the region of the internal capsule with a tumor to normal brain ratio (TBR) of 6.07 (TBR cut-off for PCNSL >2 [1]) (Fig. 3). The whole-body scan excluded the presence of systemic disease (Fig. 3). A biopsy was conducted, and the final diagnosis was a primary diffuse large B-cell lymphoma of the central nervous system. Chemotherapy was started according to R-BAM scheme (carmustine, methotrexate, cytarabine, rituximab), followed by autologous hematopoietic stem cell transplantation. Brain FDG-PET performed 6 months later showed a tumoral complete response and normalization of brain metabolism (Fig. 4), and 10 months after the clinical diagnosis, the patient was neurologically asymptomatic.

J. Arbizu (✉) · J. F. Bastidas
Department of Nuclear Medicine, Clinica Universidad de Navarra, University of Navarra, Pamplona, Spain
e-mail: jarbizu@unav.es



A. Varrone et al. (eds.), *Clinical Nuclear Medicine in Neurology*,
https://doi.org/10.1007/978-3-030-83598-9_29

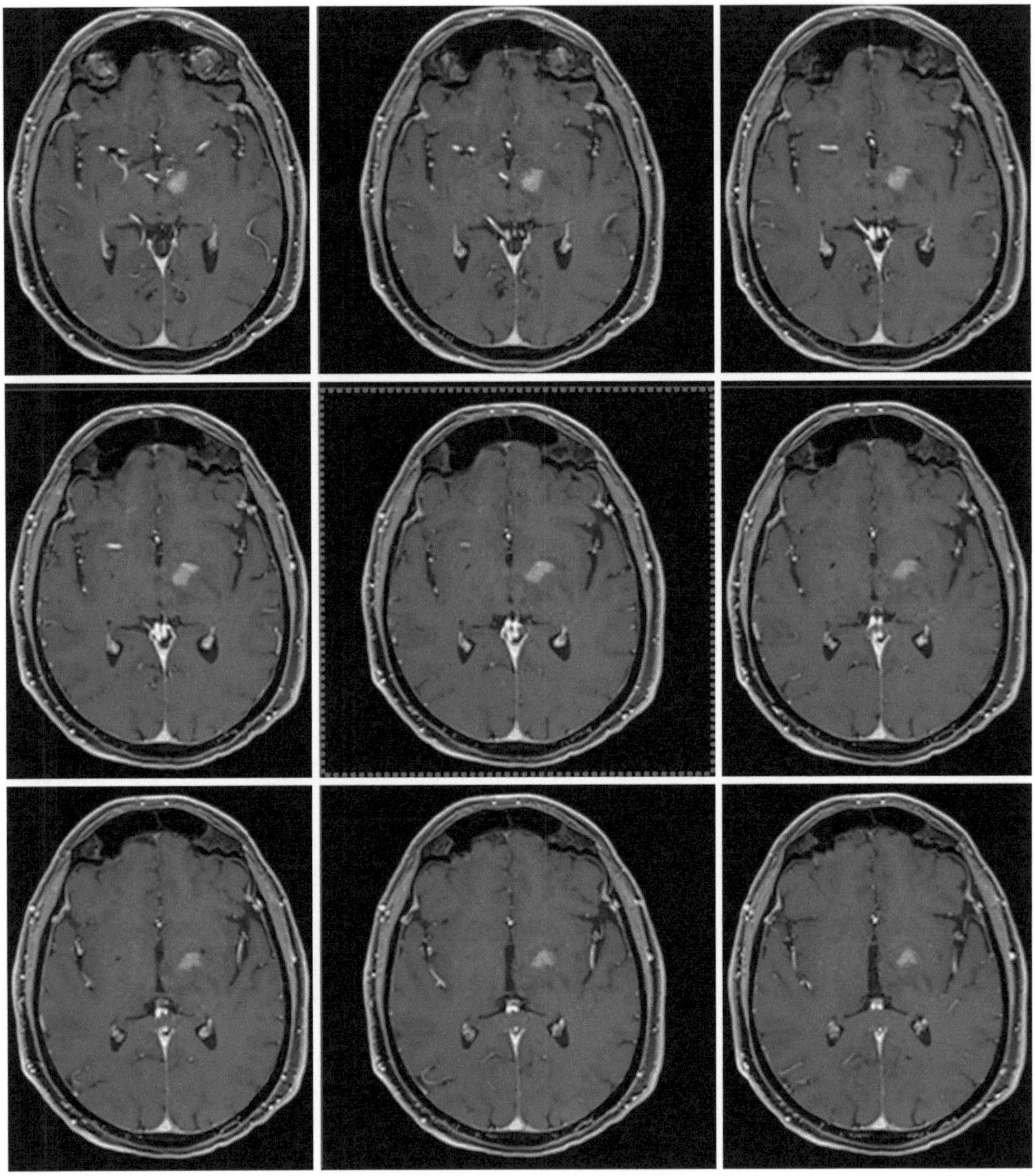

**Fig. 1** Brain MRI findings. Sequential axial series of T1 with gadolinium showing a focal area of contrast enhancement without a clear area of necrosis

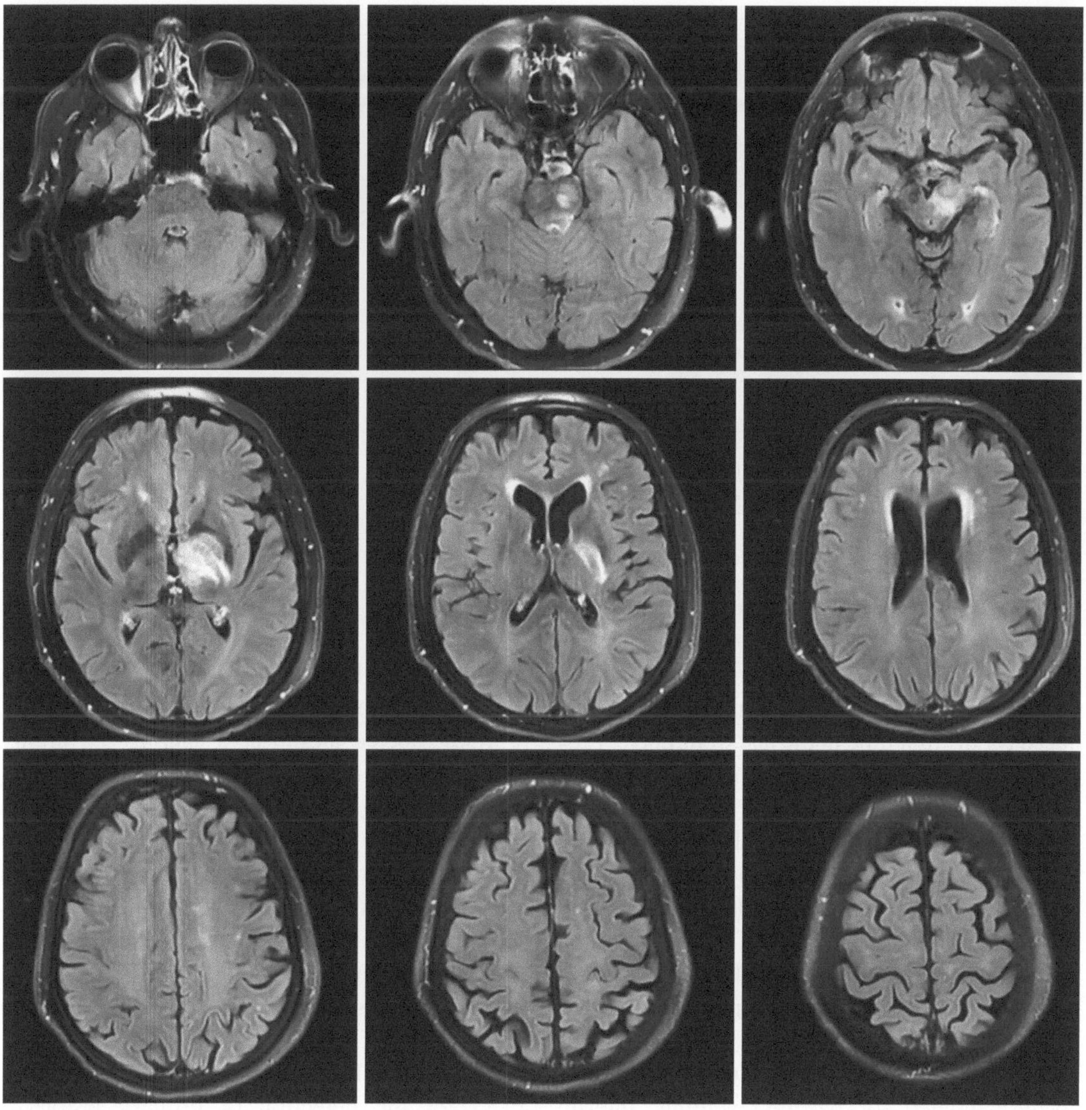

**Fig. 2** Brain MRI findings. Sequential axial series of T2 Flair showing a hypointense lesion surrounded by an area of hyperintensity

## Diagnosis

Primary diffuse large B-cell lymphoma of the central nervous system.

## Discussion

Primary central nervous system lymphoma (PCNSL), are extranodal malignant lymphomas that arise within the brain parenchyma, eyes, leptomeninges, and spinal cord in the absence of a systemic lymphoma at the time of the diagnosis [2]. It is a rare disease that accounts for 3–4% of all primary brain tumors and 4–6% of extranodal lymphomas [3]. In the past decades, the incidence data has been increasing in the immunocompetent population, while the incidence seems to be decreasing in patients with acquired immunodeficiency syndrome [2, 4]. Early diagnosis is crucial for proper management and visibility of the tumor is essential to ensure an early brain biopsy and histological diagnosis [4]. Interestingly, an expansion of entities included in

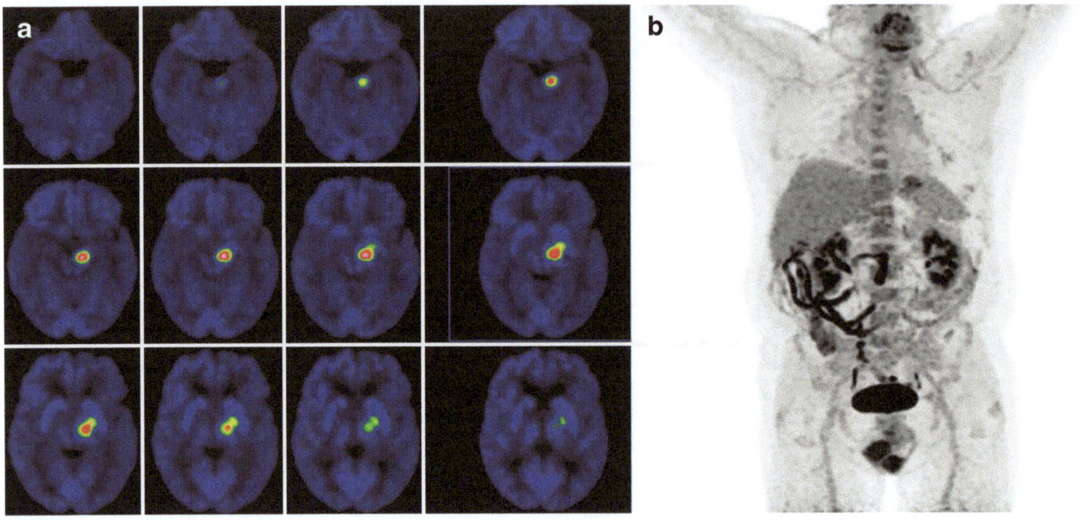


**Fig. 3** PET/CT scan with [$^{18}$F]FDG. (A) Sequential brain axial series showing an hypermetabolism on the lesion located on the left mesencephalon extending from the cerebral peduncle toward the thalamus and region of the internal capsule. (B) Whole-body scan excluding systemic disease

hematopoietic/lymphoid tumors of the CNS (lymphomas and histiocytic tumors) was introduced for the first time in the last Central Nervous System World Health Organization classification published in 2016.

An initial evaluation for the diagnosis of PCNSL involves brain MRI; in fact, due to the similar appearance on the standard MRI images between PCNSL, high-grade glioma, brain metastases, and inflammatory diseases, it could be difficult to establish the differential diagnosis.

Therefore, another supportive imaging technique is required. The use of FDG-PET is extensively validated for baseline staging, interim response assessment, and post-therapy evaluation in systemic Hodgkin lymphoma and extracranial NHL. However, it has not been systematically used for the management of PCNSL. At this respect, the metabolic imaging with FDG-PET helps the ability to distinguish between PCNSL and high-grade glioma with similar MRI findings, because the PCNSL has an extremely high FDG uptake compared to other brain tumors [1].

Radiolabeled amino acid analogs are highly recommended PET radiotracers for the evaluation of primary brain tumors. These radiotracers exhibit advantages over FDG particularly due to their low uptake in the normal brain, which can lead to determining the tumor boundaries [5]. However, Kawase et al. compared the usefulness between [$^{11}$C]methionine (MET-PET) and FDG-PET in patients with PCNSL, detecting that the uptake of MET was significantly lower than that of FDG. MET-PET showed a high sensitivity as FDG for the detection of primary lesion of PCNSL [4]. A systematic review and meta-analysis conducted by Zou et al. showed that brain FDG-PET has a considerable accuracy in identifying PCNSL in immunocompetent patients (sensitivity: 0.88 (95% CI: 0.80–0.94), specificity: 0.86 (95% CI: 0.73–0.94), area under the curve: 0.9192), and could be a valuable molecular imaging technique for PCNSL [2].

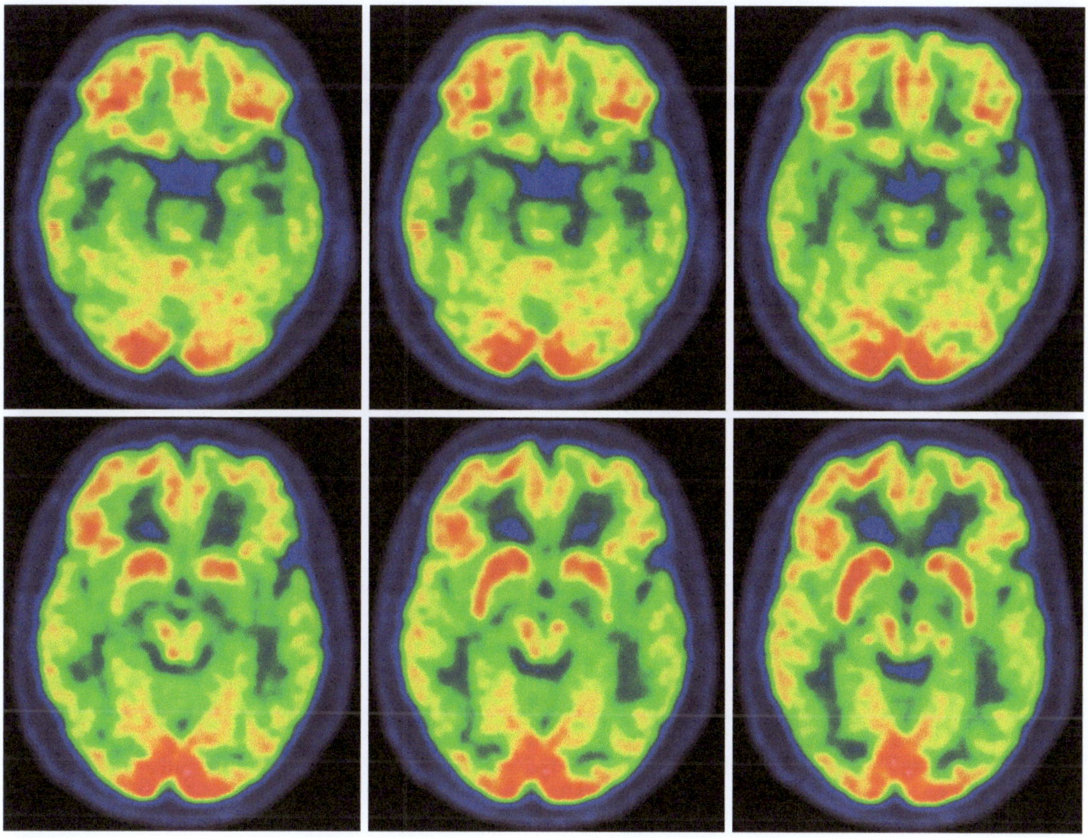

**Fig. 4** PET/CT with [$^{18}$F]FDG. Sequential axial series showing tumoral complete response and normalization of brain metabolism

## Conclusions

Brain FDG-PET can be extremely helpful for biopsy planning when PCNSL is suspected, and the lesion is located in a complex area not well defined by standard brain MRI.

Pretreatment brain FDG-PET can be included in the baseline evaluation of PCNSL not only for exclusion of systemic disease but also for further therapy assessment.

## References

1. Yamaguchi S, Hirata K, Kobayashi H, Shiga T, Manabe O, Kobayashi K, et al. The diagnostic role of 18F-FDG PET for primary central nervous system lymphoma. Ann Nucl Med. 2014;28(7):603–9.
2. Zou Y, Tong J, Leng H, Jiang J, Pan M, Chen Z. Diagnostic value of using 18F-FDG PET and PET/CT in immunocompetent patients with primary central nervous system lymphoma: a systematic review and meta-analysis. Oncotarget. 2017;8(25):41518–28.
3. Kasenda B, Haug V, Schorb E, Fritsch K, Finke J, Mix M, et al. 18F-FDG PET is an independent outcome predictor in primary central nervous system lymphoma. J Nucl Med. 2013;54(2):184–91.
4. Kawase Y, Yamamoto Y, Kameyama R, Kawai N, Kudomi N, Nishiyama Y. Comparison of 11C-methionine PET and 18F-FDG PET in patients with primary central nervous system lymphoma. Mol Imaging Biol. 2011;13(6):1284–9.
5. Ogawa T, Inugami A, Hatazawa J, Kanno I, Murakami M, Yasui N, et al. Clinical positron emission tomography for brain tumors: comparison of fludeoxyglucose F 18 and L-methyl-11C-methionine. Am J Neuroradiol. 1996;17(2):345–53.

# Case 30: Neurolymphomatosis

Tatiana Horowitz and Eric Guedj

## Case Summary

A 66-year-old man with previous history of B-cell non-Hodgkin's primary cerebral lymphoma presented for years later with intercostal neuralgia and back pain. Recent brain MRI and brain [$^{18}$F]FDG PET-CT did not show signs of relapse. Dorsal MRI and whole-body [$^{18}$F]FDG PET-CT revealed nerve lesions suspected to be a neurolymphoma, with no other remote lesions, confirmed by biopsy. CSF study showed leptomeningeal dissemination. Patient recovered after a second-line chemotherapy association.

A 66-year-old man with intercostals neuralgia and back pain (Figs. 1, 2, and 3).

Brain PET-CT was negative. Patient recovered after second-line chemotherapy.

## Epidemiology

- Highly rare cause of infiltrative neuropathy, often misdiagnosed.

T. Horowitz · E. Guedj (✉)
Aix Marseille Univ, APHM, CNRS, Centrale Marseille, Institut Fresnel, Timone Hospital, CERIMED, Nuclear Medicine Department, Marseille, France
e-mail: eric.guedj@univ-amu.fr

## Pathology and Cause

- Infiltration of cranial and peripheral nerves by a lymphoproliferative neoplasm.
- Can be the first manifestation of a lymphoma, or a site of relapse.
- Can be associated with brain or cerebrospinal fluid involvement.

## Clinical Features

- Protean manifestations depending on location: sensorimotor peripheral or cranial nerve deficits, painful neuropathy.
- Histopathological proof is often necessary.

## Clinical Management

- Radiation therapy can be attempted with risks of radiation-induced neuropathy.
- Chemotherapy sometimes in combination with rituximab can be used.

## Imaging Findings

- MRI shows nerve enlargement hyperintense in T2 and STIR sequences, enhanced after gadolinium injection.


A. Varrone et al. (eds.), *Clinical Nuclear Medicine in Neurology*,
https://doi.org/10.1007/978-3-030-83598-9_30

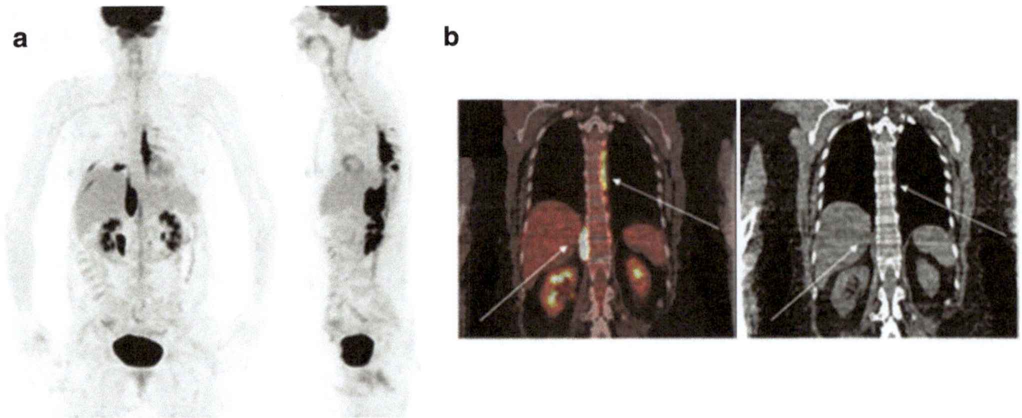

**Fig. 1** (**a**) [$^{18}$F]FDG Maximal intensity projection face and profile, and (**b**) frontal fused PET-CT and CT slices showing multifocal nerve hypermetabolic lesions, suggestive of neurolymphomatosis

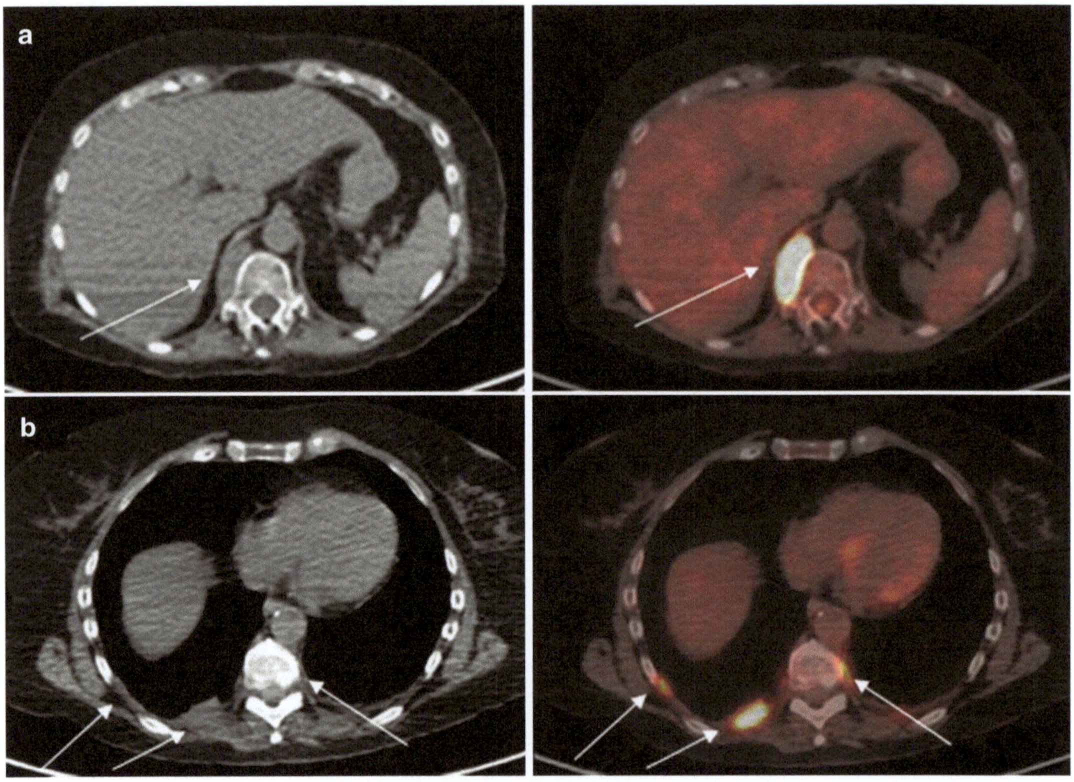

**Fig. 2** Axial fused PET-CT and CT images showing intense [$^{18}$F]FDG uptake of (**a**) right paravertebral sympathetic nerve enlargement and of (**b**) multifocal intercostals nerve lesions

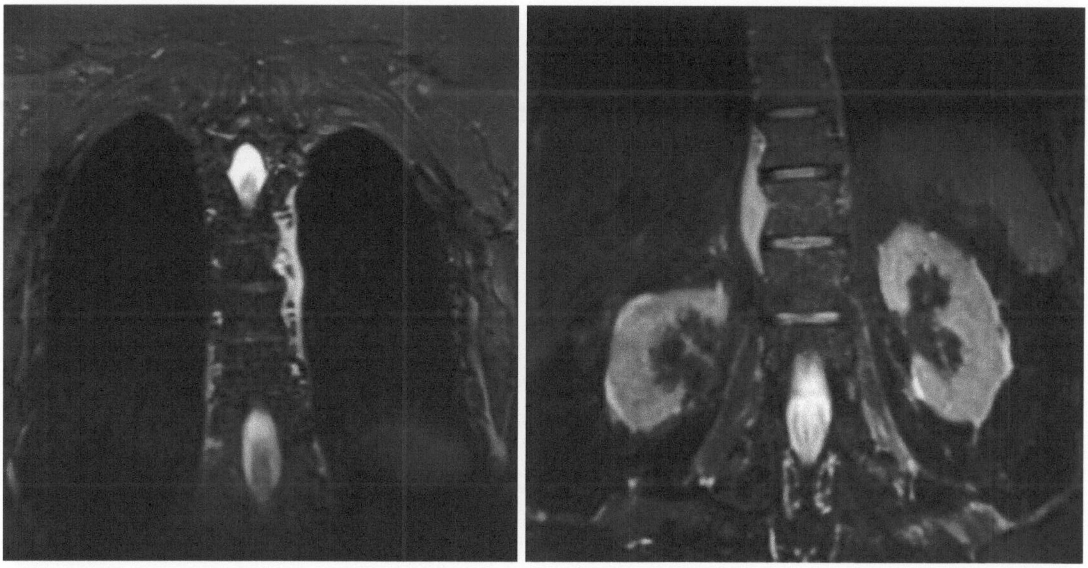

**Fig. 3** MRI STIR-weighted corresponding frontal images showing bilateral paravertebral nerves enlargement and pathological STIR hyperintensity. STIR stands for short-T1 inversion recovery and is used to null the signal from fat

- [$^{18}$F]FDG PET-CT is useful for whole-body exploration and shows intense FDG uptakes of nerve lesions.

**Take-Home Message**

- Whole-body [$^{18}$F]FDG PET-CT is the imaging modality with the highest sensibility for the detection of neurolymphomatosis.

## Further Reading

Baehring JM, Damek D, Martin EC, Betensky RA, Hochberg FH. Neurolymphomatosis. Neuro-Oncology. 2003 Apr;5(2):104–15.

Gan HK, Azad A, Cher L, Mitchell PL. Neurolymphomatosis: diagnosis, management, and outcomes in patients treated with rituximab. Neuro-Oncology. 2010;12(2):212–5.

# Case 31: Atypical Teratoid Rhabdoid Tumor (ATRT): Identification of Altered Cerebrospinal Fluid Circulation Impacting Intrathecal Chemotherapy

Tatjana Traub-Weidinger, Amedeo A. Azizi, Christian Dorfer, and Julia Furtner

## Epidemiology

Atypical teratoid rhabdoid tumor (ATRT) is a rare, aggressive, and malignant type of embryonal tumor of the central nervous system (CNS) with an incidence rate of 0.07 per 100,000 children 0–19 years old, occurring most often in children younger than 3 years old [1]. ATRT constitutes 20% of all CNS tumors in this population and up to 50% in infants below 1 year of age [2]. Described for the first time as a distinct type of CNS rhabdoid tumor in 1987 [3], this tumor entity was later implemented in the World Health Organization (WHO) classification of CNS tumors in 2000. INI1 loss is seen as a hallmark of ATRT [2]. Recently, three main distinct molecular subtypes of ATRT have been described [4]. Occurring anywhere in the CNS, supratentorial tumors are more common with increasing age [1]. In 20–40% of cases, metastatic spread has already occured at presentation. In a high number of cases, ATRT occurs on the background of a rhabdoid tumor syndrome with germline SMARCB1 or SMARCA4 loss [2]. Until now, there is no consensus regarding an established and standardized therapy. A complete surgical resection can often be challenging but should be attempted if safely feasible. Different chemotherapy regimens have been investigated, often including high-dose chemotherapy and intrathecal chemotherapy (i.e., application of chemotherapeutic agents directly into the cerebrospinal fluid (CSF)). Radiotherapy (focal or craniospinal) is included in many therapeutic approaches and seems to enhance survival [2]. Prognosis generally remains poor, with 5-year overall survival (OS) rates of approximately 35%, whereas some treatment regimens (e.g., MUV-ATRT) may reach higher OS rates [5, 6].

One feature of this tumor entity is disturbance of cerebrospinal fluid (CSF) flow by either metastases or rapid tumor growth causing ventricular obstruction over a short period of time. Therefore, patients may need emergency surgical decompression treat-

T. Traub-Weidinger (✉)
Division of Nuclear Medicine, Department of Biomedical Imaging and Image-Guided Therapy, Medical University of Vienna, Vienna, Austria
e-mail: tatjana.traub-weidinger@meduniwien.ac.at

A. A. Azizi
Department of Pediatrics and Adolescent Medicine, Medical University of Vienna, Vienna, Austria

C. Dorfer
Department of Neurosurgery, Medical University of Vienna, Vienna, Austria

J. Furtner
Division of Neuro- and Musculoskeletal Radiology, Department of Biomedical imaging and Image-guided Therapy, Medical University of Vienna, Vienna, Austria


A. Varrone et al. (eds.), *Clinical Nuclear Medicine in Neurology*,
https://doi.org/10.1007/978-3-030-83598-9_31

ment of intracranial hypertension and/or hydrocephalus by ventricular drainage. Drug delivery systems such as Ommaya or Rickham Reservoirs are required for the intrathecal therapeutic management of these patients.

## Imaging Techniques

Computed tomography (CT) and magnetic resonance imaging (MRI) are the gold-standard in the diagnosis and follow-up of brain tumors. Besides tumor-related details, these techniques are also important to reveal tumor-independent information regarding treatment-associated complications such as hemorrhage or infarction, malposition of catheters or signs of increased intracranial pressure due to an obstruction of the cerebrospinal fluid (CSF) circulation.

Cerebrospinal fluid (CSF) scintigraphy (also referred to as "cisternogram") is a traditional clinical nuclear medicine neuroimaging modality, in former times helpful in diagnosing normal pressure hydrocephalus (NPH), nowadays mostly used to detect CSF leaks or to evaluate CSF shunt patency and sites of possible obstruction, which is important to know for intrathecal treatment planning. This nuclear medicine procedure is a simple, effective, and low-radiation-dose method for assessing CSF flow and a useful tool in the management of patients presenting shunt-related or CNS obstruction problems not elucidated by conventional radiological examination.

## Clinical History

A 6-month-old male infant was admitted to the hospital with vomiting and altered vigilance as signs of elevated intracranial pressure (ICP). MR imaging revealed an avid contrast-enhancing mass in the third ventricle arising from the mesencephalon, which consecutively led to an obstructive hydrocephalus (*See* Fig. 1). The hydrocephalus was relieved by a neurosurgically placed extra-ventricular drainage (EVD). The tumor was then surgically removed, and an EVD was replaced for a few days after the tumor operation. The patient developed bilateral hygroma, and after the removal of the EVD, the patient needed placement of a subduro-peritoneal shunt (i.e., a connection between the hygroma and the peritoneal cavity). Histology revealed an ATRT and treatment was started with intravenous chemotherapy according to MUV-ATRT protocol [6]. In order to allow intrathecal chemotherapy (ith. CTX), an Ommaya reservoir was placed to allow the antineoplastic drugs to spread in the CSF space. The tip of the catheter was correctly located at the bottom of the third ventricle (*See* Fig. 2).

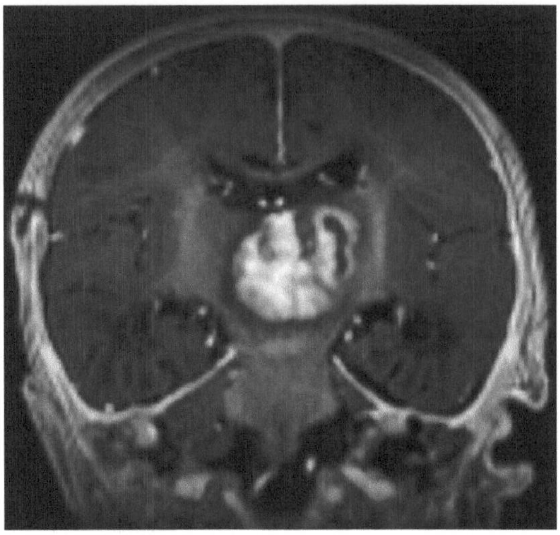

**Fig. 1** Coronar T1-weighted contrast-enhanced MR images of a mass in the third ventricle, which was histopathologically diagnosed as an ATRT

As CSF circulation with bilateral hygroma and subduro-peritoneal shunt dependency and consecutively also the intrathecal drug distribution was uncertain, Indium 111-labeled diethylene triamine pentaacetic acid (DTPA) was applied over the Ommaya reservoir to track its distribution. Besides the Ommaya reservoir, the tracer could be only detected in the third ventricle, without entering the spinal canal or showing any tracer distribution over the cerebral convexity detected by scintigraphic imaging over 24 h, indicating a correctly working Ommaya reservoir system but a hindrance of the CSF flow to the spinal canal or over both hemispheres (*see* Fig. 3). Therefore, the subduro-peritoneal shunt

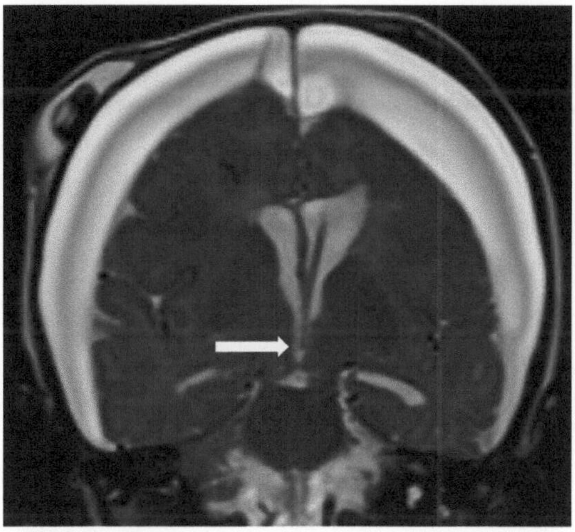

**Fig. 2** Coronar T2-weighted MRI sequence depicting the localization of the Ommaya catheter tip at the bottom of the third ventricle (white arrow)

was ligated and a Torkildson drain was implanted, connecting the right-sided ventricle and the fourth ventricle (linked via T-piece) to the spinal canal (*see* Fig. 4).

$^{111}$Indium DTPA distribution was then seen not only in the third ventricle but also in the spinal canal and over both hemispheres within 1 h after tracer application with no further obstruction of flow over the following 24 h. Only a difference in tracer activity over the convexities was still observed caused by hygroma presentation (*see* Fig. 5). Due to CSF leakage, ith. CTX has to be halted after a few weeks, and the ligation of the subduro-peritoneal shunt had to be removed, thereby re-opening the shunt. At the same time, an on/off device was placed, allowing temporary

**Fig. 3** Planar images (posterior views) 1 h and 24 h (from right to left) after In111 DTPA administration over the Ommaya reservoir showing persistence of tracer activity in the ventricular system. Tracer was observed over both hemispheres but not in the spinal canal

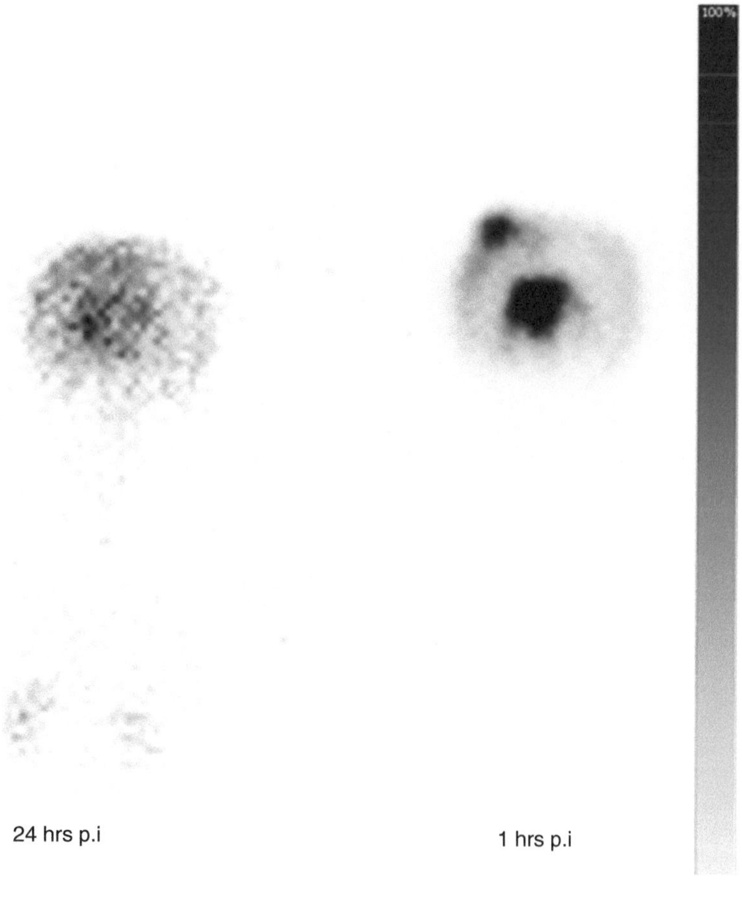

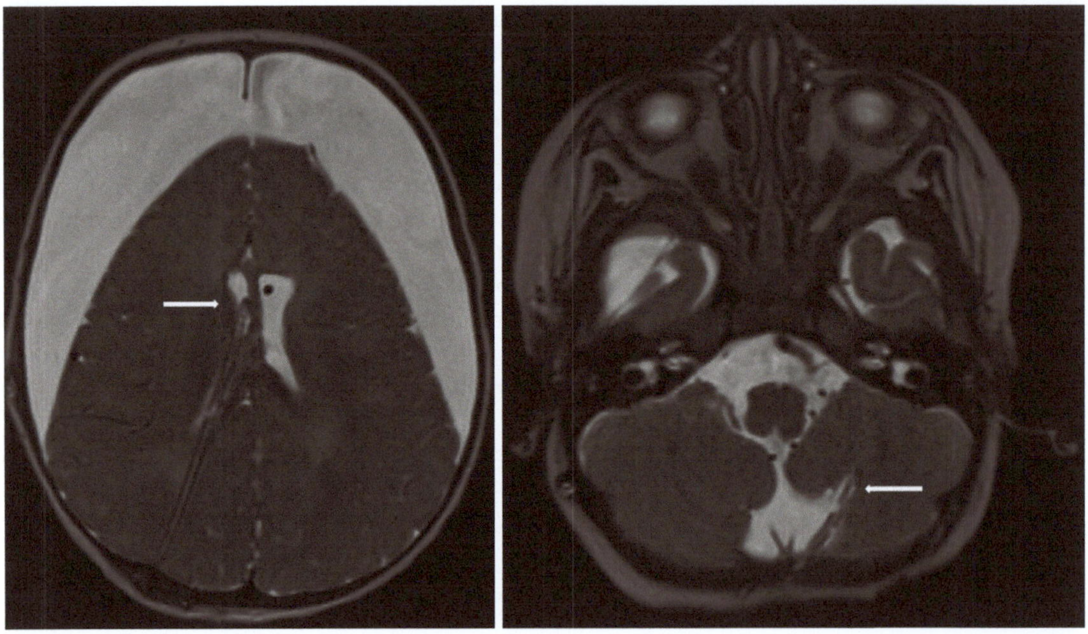

**Fig. 4** Axial T2-weighted MR images depicting the tip of the Torkildson drain in the right-sided ventricle (A) and the left-sided subarachnoid CSF space in the inferior posterior portion of the posterior fossa (B) (white arrow)

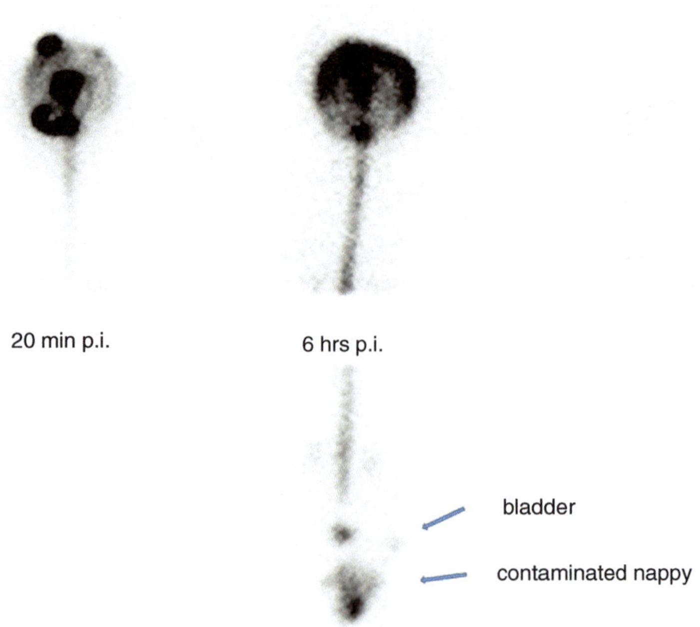


**Fig. 5** Planar images (posterior views) 20 min, 6 h, and 24 h of the second [$^{111}$In]DTPA scintigraphy with tracer application to the Ommaya reservoir showing rapid tracer distribution over the convexity and to the spinal canal with persistence of the tracer over 24 h without any hindrance of flow

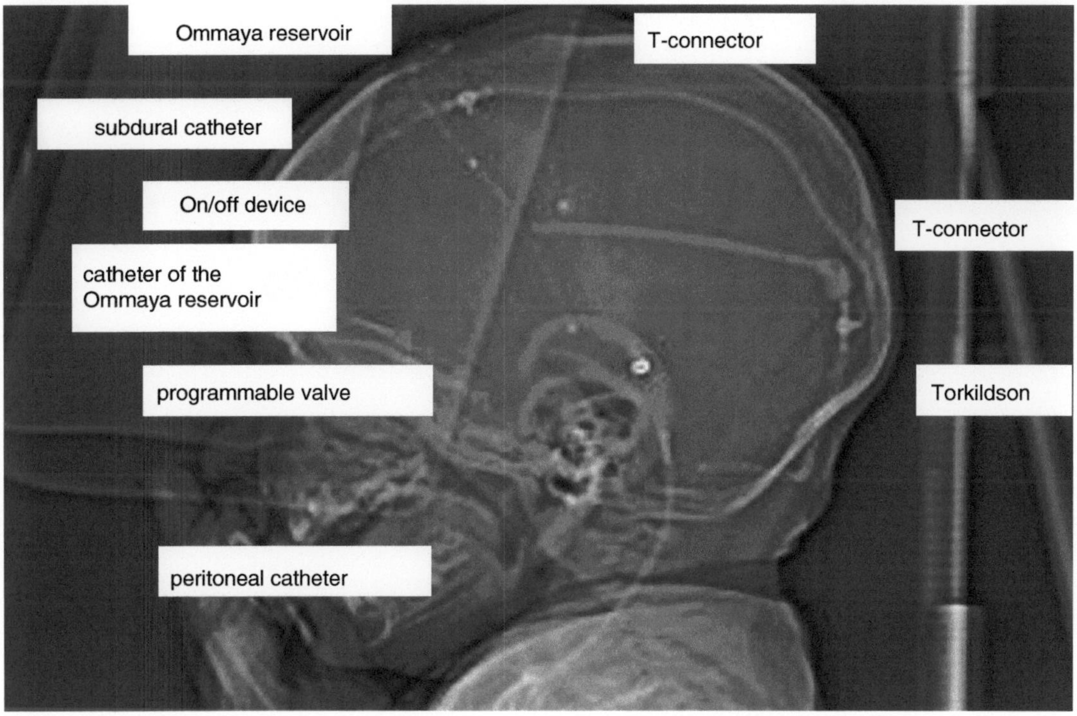


**Fig. 6** X-ray of the head giving an overview of all implanted CSF catheters and devices

occlusion of the shunt system (usually for a few hours) after the application of ith. CTX in order to enhance CSF circulation of the drug and slow its drainage into the peritoneal cavity (*see* Fig. 6).

Nevertheless, the patient developed a metastatic tumor spread 6 months after initial diagnosis. Therapy was therefore switched to an antiangiogenic treatment according to MEMMAT protocol [7]. A newly conducted Indium-DTPA scan revealed insufficient tracer distribution to the spinal canal once again (*see* Fig. 7). Therefore, ith. CTX was extended by intralumbar application of a long-lasting liposomal cytarabine formulation [8]. Despite intensive treatment, the tumor spread worsened and the patient deteriorated clinically, developing untreatable BNS-like seizures, dysphagia, and aspiration pneumonia. The patient received palliative care and finally succumbed to his disease less than a year after the diagnosis of his ATRT.

## Closing Remarks

Intrathecal drug delivery systems have become widely used and established tools in the management of refractory chronic pain and spasticity as well as in oncology. Suspicion of possible mechanical complications related to the implanted

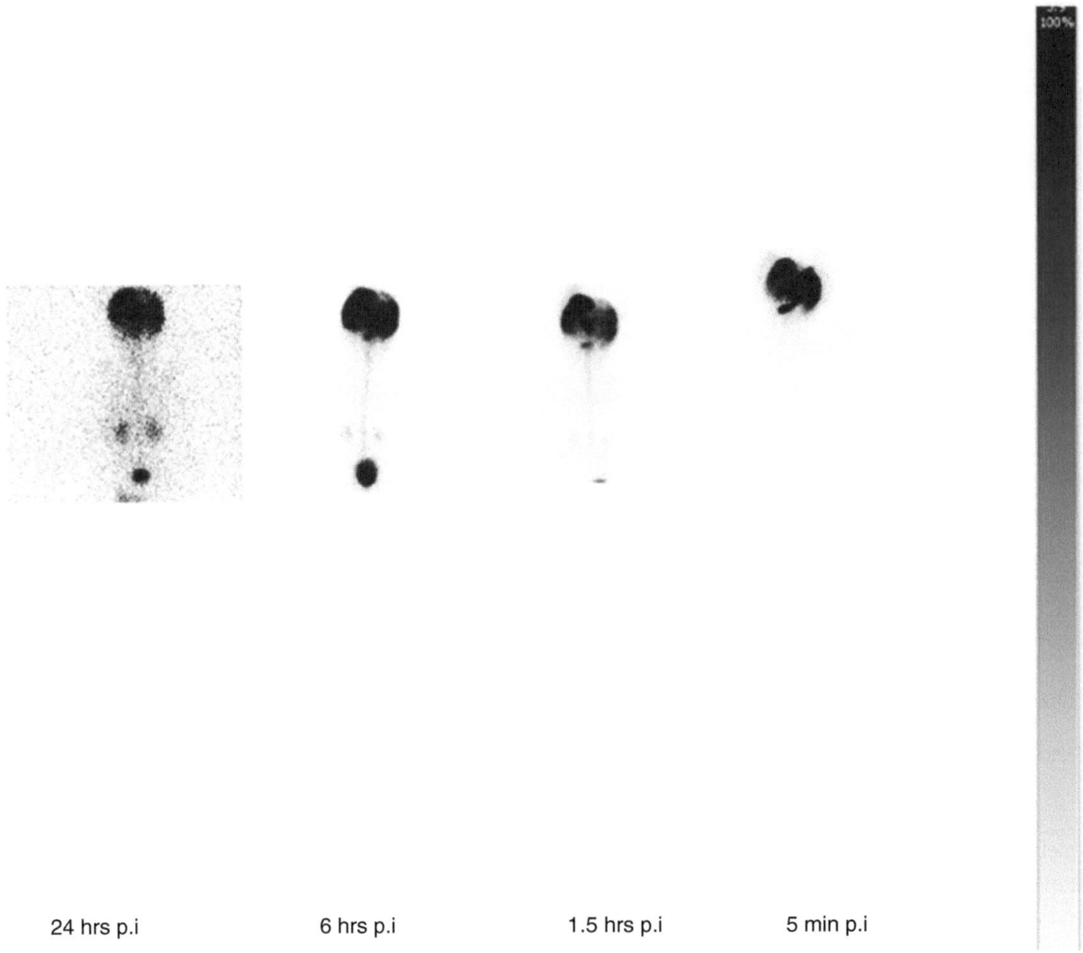


**Fig. 7** Planar images (posterior views) 5 min, 1.5 h, 6 h, and 24 h (from right to left) after the third [$^{111}$In]DTPA administration to the Ommaya reservoir showing a quite rapid tracer distribution over the convexity but only a poor tracer accumulation in the spinal canal

system or changes in the CSF flow due to disease progression often necessitates further investigations. This, however, may present a diagnostic challenge. CSF scintigraphy is a useful, low-radiation-dose imaging tool for functional verification of CSF flow and allows verification of the patency of a CSF shunt or intrathecal medical drug delivery systems as well as of drug distribution in the CSF space over time.

## References

1. Ostrom QT, Chen Y, de Blank PM, Ondracek A, Farah P, Gittleman H, Wolinsky Y, Kruchko C, Cohen ML, Brat DJ, Barnholtz-Sloan JS. The descriptive epidemiology of atypical teratoid/rhabdoid tumors in the United States, 2001–2010 Quinn T. Neuro-Oncology. 2014;16(10):1392–9. https://doi.org/10.1093/neuonc/nou090.
2. Nesvick CL, Lafay-Cousin L, Raghunathan A, Bouffet E, Huang AA, Daniels DJ. Atypical teratoid rhabdoid

tumor: molecular insights and translation to novel therapeutics. J Neuro-Oncol. 2020 Oct;150(1):47–56. https://doi.org/10.1007/s11060-020-03639-w.

3. Lefkowitz IB, Rorke JB, Packer R, Sutton LN, Siegel KR, Katnick RJ. Atypical teratoid tumor of infancy: definition of an entity. Ann Neurol. 1987;22(3):448–9.
4. Ho B, Johann PD, Grabovska Y, De Dieu Andrianteranagna MJ, Yao F, Frühwald M, Hasselblatt M, Bourdeaut F, Williamson D, Huang A, Kool M. Molecular subgrouping of atypical teratoid/rhabdoid tumors-a reinvestigation and current consensus. Neuro-Oncology. 2020 May 15;22(5):613–24. https://doi.org/10.1093/neuonc/noz235.
5. Frühwald MC, Hasselblatt M, Nemes K, Bens S, Steinbügl M, Johann PD, Kerl K, Hauser P, Quiroga E, Solano-Paez P, Biassoni V, Gil-da-Costa MJ, Perek-Polnik M, van de Wetering M, Sumerauer D, Pears J, Stabell N, Holm S, Hengartner H, Gerber NU, Grotzer M, Boos J, Ebinger M, Tippelt S, Paulus W, Furtwängler R, Hernáiz-Driever P, Reinhard H, Rutkowski S, Schlegel PG, Schmid I, Kortmann RD, Timmermann B, Warmuth-Metz M, Kordes U, Gerss J, Nysom K, Schneppenheim R, Siebert R, Kool M, Graf N. Age and DNA methylation subgroup as potential independent risk factors for treatment stratification in children with atypical teratoid/rhabdoid tumors. Neuro-Oncology. 2020 Jul 7;22(7):1006–17. https://doi.org/10.1093/neuonc/noz244.
6. Slavc I, Chocholous M, Leiss U, Haberler C, Peyrl A, Azizi AA, Dieckmann K, Woehrer A, Peters C, Widhalm G, Dorfer C, Czech T. Atypical teratoid rhabdoid tumor: improved long-term survival with an intensive multimodal therapy and delayed radiotherapy. The Medical University of Vienna experience 1992-2012. Cancer Med. 2014 Feb;3(1):91–100. https://doi.org/10.1002/cam4.161.
7. Peyrl A, Chocholous M, Kieran MW, Azizi AA, Prucker C, Czech T, Dieckmann K, Schmook MT, Haberler C, Leiss U, Slavc I. Antiangiogenic metronomic therapy for children with recurrent embryonal brain tumors. Pediatr Blood Cancer. 2012 Sep;59(3):511–7. https://doi.org/10.1002/pbc.24006.
8. Peyrl A, Sauermann R, Chocholous M, Azizi AA, Jäger W, Höferl M, Slavc I. Pharmacokinetics and toxicity of intrathecal liposomal cytarabine in children and adolescents following age-adapted dosing. Clin Pharmacokinet. 2014 Feb;53(2):165–73. https://doi.org/10.1007/s40262-013-0106-1.

# Case 32: Suspected Recurrence of Brain Metastasis After Radiotherapy

Marcus Unterrainer, Adrien Holzgreve, Bogdana Suchorska, and Nathalie L. Albert

A 64-year-old female patient presented with increasing headache and staggering vertigo. In previous medical history, the patient underwent resection and adjuvant radiochemotherapy for poorly differentiated pulmonary adenocarcinoma with oligofocal brain metastases, which were previously treated with radiosurgery and proton therapy.

For further clinical evaluation, a contrast-enhanced MRI of the brain was performed. Here, at the previous site of a brain metastasis, a large unifocal contrast-enhancing lesion at the left parasagittal lobe was seen on gadolinium-enhanced, T1-weighted MRI imaging (see Fig. 1A). The ring-enhancing lesion showed an extension of 3.2 × 1.7 × 2.7 cm with central necrosis and was accompanied by an extensive perifocal edema in the left hemisphere on T2-weighted MRI imaging (see Fig. 1B). Further contrast-enhancing lesions were not detectable. Overall, the MRI scan was highly suspicious of brain metastasis recurrence. However, as proton therapy was applied approximately 2 years previously, differential diagnosis also included extensive radionecrosis with consecutive edema.

For further evaluation, an additional dynamic amino acid PET using O-(2-$^{18}$F-fluoroethyl)-L-tyrosine ([$^{18}$F]FET) was performed. Here, only a faint circular FET uptake was noted with only moderate semi-quantitative parameters with mean and maximum tumor-to-background ratios ($TBR_{mean/max}$) of only 1.89 and 2.09, respectively, untypical findings for vital tumor masses, which usually present with extensively elevated [$^{18}$F]FET uptake on PET (see Fig. 1C with a PET image and Fig. 1D for a PET image fused to the contrast-enhanced, T1-weighted MRI). As dynamic PET also provides additional information for the differentiation of recurrent tumor masses and radionecrosis, a dynamic analysis of the PET study was performed in addition. PET images were evaluated in a slice-by-slice manner, and the minimal time-to-peak ($TTP_{min}$) was analyzed; this revealed constantly increasing time–activity curves along the contrast-enhancing

M. Unterrainer
Department of Radiology, University Hospital, LMU Munich, Munich, Germany

Department of Nuclear Medicine, University Hospital, LMU Munich, Munich, Germany
e-mail: Marcus.Unterrainer@med.uni-muenchen.de

A. Holzgreve · N. L. Albert (✉)
Department of Nuclear Medicine, University Hospital, LMU Munich, Munich, Germany
e-mail: Adrien.Holzgreve@med.uni-muenchen.de; Nathalie.Albert@med.uni-muenchen.de

B. Suchorska
Department of Neurosurgery, University Hospital, LMU Munich, Munich, Germany
e-mail: Bogdana.Suchorska@med.uni-muenchen.de


A. Varrone et al. (eds.), *Clinical Nuclear Medicine in Neurology*,
https://doi.org/10.1007/978-3-030-83598-9_32

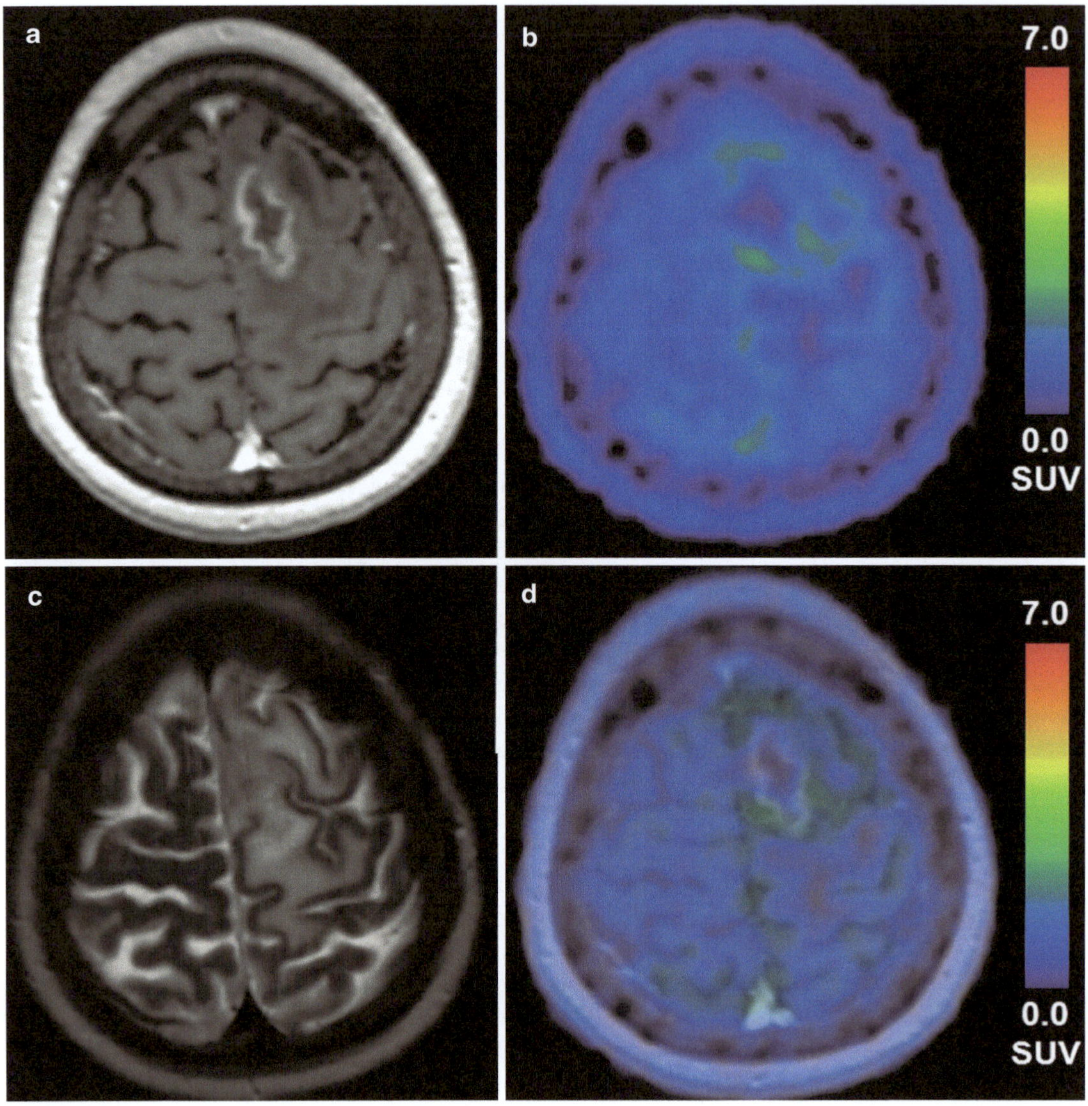


**Fig. 1** Patient example: (**a**) contrast enhanced T1 MRI, (**b**) FET PET, (**c**) T2 MRI, (**d**) fused FET PET/contrast enhanced MRI

lesion with a consecutive $TTP_{min}$ of 35 minutes, also a feature untypical for tumor recurrence (see Fig. 1E).

Due to the clinical presentation, an additional stereotactic biopsy was taken from the frontal lesion to finally confirm the PET-suspected radionecrosis. Here, only gliotic tissue with reactive astrocytes and foam cells were present, but no recurrent vital tumor tissue. Hence, the patient received anti-edematous therapy consisting of dexamethasone for the treatment of the histologically proven radionecrosis.

In clinical routine, the differentiation of recurrent brain metastases from radiation necrosis after previous radiotherapy (e.g., stereotactic radiotherapy, radiosurgery, proton therapy) can be challenging based on MRI alone, as radionecrosis can present with similar imaging features such as ring-shaped contrast enhancement and extensive perifocal edema [1], consecutively leading to clinical symptoms also comparable to those that accompany tumor recurrence. Nonetheless, noninvasive imaging techniques for the accurate differentiation of recurrent tumor and radionecrosis are desirable in clinical routine, as treatment strategies are highly diverging from anti-edematous/anti-angiogenic therapy (e.g., dexamethasone or bevacizumab [1]) and anti-tumor therapy (e.g., resection, systemic treatment) [2].

Beyond MRI, PET imaging using radiolabeled amino acids such as L-methyl-$^{11}$C-methionine ([$^{11}$C]MET), [$^{18}$F]fluoro-dihydroxyphenylalanine ([$^{18}$F]DOPA), and [$^{18}$F]FET has shown to add significant information for this clinical issue [3]. With regard to [$^{18}$F]FET PET, the additional acquisition of a dynamic study provides additional diagnostic value for the differentiation of radionecrosis [4, 5]. Although static parameters such as the $TBR_{mean}$ already enable a high accuracy for the differentiation of radiation-induced changes from viable tumor at a cut-off value of 2.0, the diagnostic power can be further increased by the implementation of dynamic information [4–6]. Therefore, despite the longer scan duration of 40 minutes, the dynamic acquisition of [$^{18}$F]FET PET should be the mode of choice whenever possible. The persistently frequent use of [$^{18}$F]fluorodeoxyglucose ([$^{18}$F]FDG) PET is of highly limited value due to a knowingly poor target-to-background contrast as well as unspecific [$^{18}$F]FDG uptake of inflammatory cells with consecutively limited diagnostic accuracy [7]. As presented in the current Response Assessment in Neuro-Oncology criteria (RANO) PET working group report on PET imaging in metastases [3], the different radiolabeled amino acids for PET imaging have shown a high accuracy for the differentiation of recurrence and radionecrosis. Moreover, more sophisticated methods for image analysis such as radiomics and deep learning approaches have shown to increase the diagnostic accuracy for this clinical issue [8, 9]. [$^{18}$F]FET PET has furthermore proven to be cost-effective when performed in addition to MRI for this clinical issue [10].

In sum, amino acid PET can significantly contribute to the clinical scenario of suspected tumor recurrence vs. treatment-related changes/radionecrosis with distinct superiority over [$^{18}$F]FDG PET.

## References


1. Le Rhun E, Dhermain F, Vogin G, Reyns N, Metellus P. Radionecrosis after stereotactic radiotherapy for brain metastases. Expert Rev Neurother. 2016;16(8):903–14.
2. Soffietti R, Abacioglu U, Baumert B, Combs SE, Kinhult S, Kros JM, et al. Diagnosis and treatment of brain metastases from solid tumors: guidelines from the European Association of Neuro-Oncology (EANO). Neuro-Oncology. 2017;19(2):162–74.
3. Galldiks N, Langen K-J, Albert NL, Chamberlain M, Soffietti R, Kim MM, et al. PET imaging in patients with brain metastasis—report of the RANO/PET group. Neuro-Oncology. 2019;21(5):585–95.
4. Ceccon G, Lohmann P, Stoffels G, Judov N, Filss CP, Rapp M, et al. Dynamic O-(2-18F-fluoroethyl)-L-tyrosine positron emission tomography differentiates brain metastasis recurrence from radiation injury after radiotherapy. Neuro-Oncology. 2017;19(2):281–8.
5. Romagna A, Unterrainer M, Schmid-Tannwald C, Brendel M, Tonn J-C, Nachbichler SB, et al. Suspected recurrence of brain metastases after focused high dose radiotherapy: can [18 F] FET-PET overcome diagnostic uncertainties? Radiat Oncol. 2016;11(1):139.
6. Galldiks N, Stoffels G, Filss CP, Piroth MD, Sabel M, Ruge MI, et al. Role of O-(2-18F-fluoroethyl)-L-tyrosine PET for differentiation of local recurrent brain metastasis from radiation necrosis. J Nucl Med. 2012;53(9):1367–74.
7. Diaz ME, Debowski M, Hukins C, Fielding D, Fong KM, Bettington CS. Non-small cell lung cancer brain metastasis screening in the era of positron emission tomography-CT staging: current practice and outcomes. J Med Imaging Radiat Oncol. 2018;62(3):383–8.
8. Lohmann P, Kocher M, Ceccon G, Bauer EK, Stoffels G, Viswanathan S, et al. Combined FET PET/MRI radiomics differentiates radiation injury from recurrent brain metastasis. NeuroImage: Clinical. 2018;20:537–42.
9. Lohmann P, Stoffels G, Ceccon G, Rapp M, Sabel M, Filss CP, et al. Radiation injury vs. recurrent brain metastasis: combining textural feature radiomics analysis and standard parameters may increase 18 F-FET PET accuracy without dynamic scans. Eur Radiol. 2017;27(7):2916–27.
10. Heinzel A, Müller D, Yekta-Michael SS, Ceccon G, Langen K-J, Mottaghy FM, et al. O-(2-18F-fluoroethyl)-L-tyrosine PET for evaluation of brain metastasis recurrence after radiotherapy: an effectiveness and cost-effectiveness analysis. Neuro-Oncology. 2017;19(9):1271–8.

# Case 33: Tumefactive Multiple Sclerosis Lesions (TMS)

Silvia Morbelli and Stefano Raffa

## Introduction

Multiple sclerosis (MS) is an immune-mediated progressive inflammatory disease affecting myelinated axons in the central nervous system (CNS), destroying myelin and axon at various levels and producing physical disability. Diagnosis of MS involves careful assessment of medical history, neurological examination, magnetic resonance imaging (T2-weighted MRI with emphasis on the spatial and temporal distribution of lesions) of the brain and spine, and cerebrospinal fluid analysis.

Tumefactive multiple sclerosis (TMS) is a rarer variant of MS that poses a diagnostic challenge, as it can be difficult to differentiate these types of lesions from CNS neoplasia or other types of CNS lesions. In fact, these lesions mimic a brain tumor clinically, radiologically, and even pathologically in some cases. Tumefactive demyelinating lesions (TDLs) are generally defined as acute, large (>2 cm), tumor-like demyelinating lesions in the CNS that occur with surrounding edema, mass effect, and ring enhancement.

The incidence and prevalence of demyelinating swelling lesions are 1–3/1000 and 0.3/100,000, respectively, with a prevalence in females compared to males (3:1 in most studies).

TDLs are likely related to various disorders in the framework of demyelinating, infective, autoimmune, paraneoplastic, and drug-induced diseases.

The clinical presentation is often characterized by predominance of cortical signs although other signs and symptoms may occur.

Surrounding edema and mass effect are generally visible, less intense than primary brain tumors at MRI. Similarly, the enhancement of the ring, if present, is mostly incomplete and open to the cortex (with the enhancement portion believed to represent the anterior border of demyelination pointing to the white matter side of the lesion). Low regional cerebral blood flow (rCBF) and regional brain blood volume (rCBV) tend to be present as TDLs do not show clear neovascularization. N-acetylaspartate (NAA) and increased choline peak can be present.

Some peculiar features of MRI can lead to a correct diagnosis, particularly with respect to high-grade neoplasm. However, MRI perfusion imaging may not be conclusive in some cases due to the variability of brain blood volume characterizing several tumor types, including primary CNS lymphoma.

S. Morbelli (✉) · S. Raffa
IRCCS Ospedale Policlinico San Martino, Genoa, Italy

Nuclear Medicine Unit, Department of Health Sciences, University of Genoa, Genoa, Italy
e-mail: silviadaniela.morbelli@hsanmartino.it


A. Varrone et al. (eds.), *Clinical Nuclear Medicine in Neurology*,
https://doi.org/10.1007/978-3-030-83598-9_33

Increasing the accuracy of imaging for the identification of TDL is of interest to avoid more invasive procedure such as brain biopsy.

[$^{18}$F]FDG is the most widely used tracer in oncology; however, its role is limited in neuro-oncology due to the high physiological uptake at cortical level. Accordingly, PET imaging of tracers able to track amino-acid (AA) uptake (AA PET) have been proposed in this clinical setting.

The majority of the few small studies or cases series on the use of AA for the differential diagnosis of TDL is based on the use of [$^{11}$C] methionine (MET-PET). In these preliminary studies, MET-PET was able to noninvasively diagnose TMS by demonstrating moderate or absent tracer uptake in lesions mimicking glioblastoma on MRI. Case reports or small case series showing PET imaging in patients with tumefactive plaques have to-date been published using other tracers for amino acid imaging such as [$^{18}$F]fluoroethyl-L-tyrosine (FET). To date, no data of patients with TMS who underwent PET imaging with 18F-Dopa are available. Although, at least in principle, we should expect similar findings with respect to what is previously evident for MET and FET-PET, [$^{18}$F]fluorodopa might have some peculiar features of interest in this settings (i.e., the capability to compare uptake with the physiological uptake of the basal ganglia).

## Case Presentation

- A 71-year-old woman with relapse and remission MS originally diagnosed 15 years earlier.
- Several different therapies have been administered in the course of years of disease: interferon beta 1a, natalizumab, glatiramer acetate had been administered.
- Before 2 years, a bilateral breast cancer was also diagnosed and treated with surgery and chemotherapy.
- After 2 years characterized by substantial absence of focal symptoms, she showed acute onset Aphasia, and she was submitted to MRI.

## Imaging Findings

MRI documenting new bilateral areas of altered hyperintense signal in the T2-weighted and hypointense sequences in T1-weighted images. Lesions were characterized by contrast enhancement with a complete peripheral ring in the temporo-parieto-occipital in the right hemisphere and in the frontal cortex in the left hemisphere.

- A differential diagnosis (especially for the left frontal lesion) was proposed between TDL and metastatic lesions (which were considered also given patient's previous history of oncologic disease, Fig. 1).
- Given the need to support this differential diagnosis avoiding brain biopsy, [$^{18}$F]fluorodopa PET was performed. PET examination demonstrates mild-to-moderate uptake only in the peripheral part of the larger lesion in the left lateral frontal (SUVr with the striatum 0.6). Even milder uptake was also observed in two lesions located respectively in the left temporo-parieto-occipital area and close to the posterior horn of the left ventricle (SUVr with the striatum 0.5). The described metabolic behavior suggested the presence of TDL rather than of metastatic lesion from breast cancer (Fig. 2).
- Therapy with rituximab was thus started with symptoms remission, and a post-therapy MRI was performed 4 months later.
- MRI: The size of the lesion located in the left frontal cortex was clearly reduced while the lesion in the right temporo-parieto-occipital cortex was no longer evident (Fig. 3).

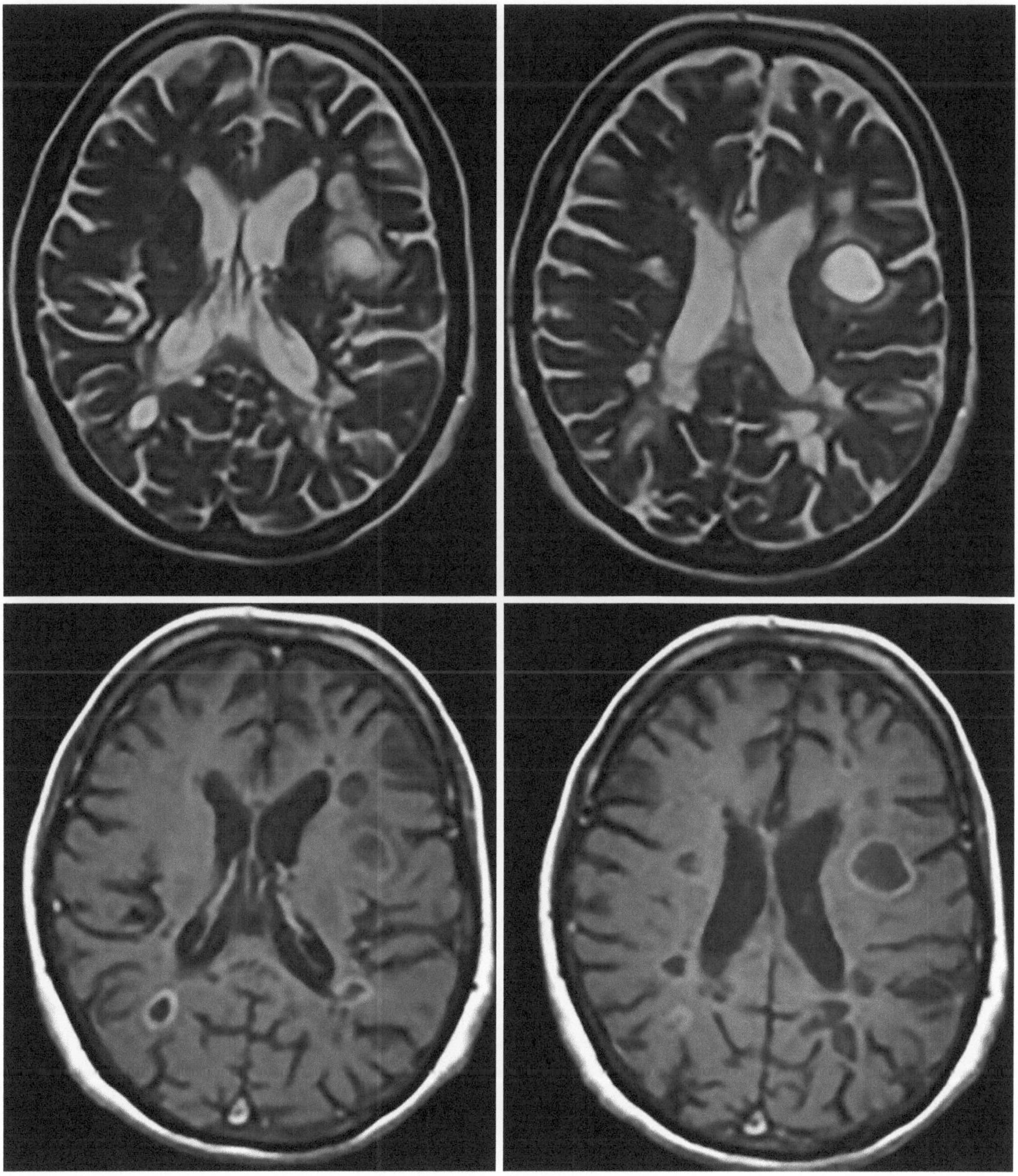

**Fig. 1** Axial brain MR T2 and gadolinium-enhanced T1-weighted images

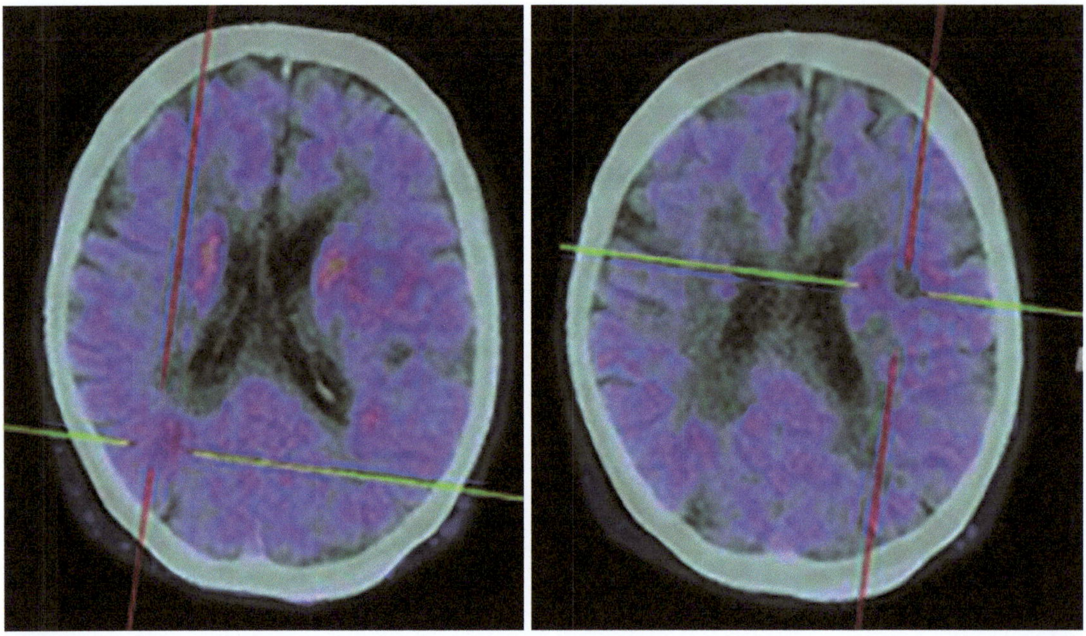

**Fig. 2** Axial images brain F-DOPA PET/CT

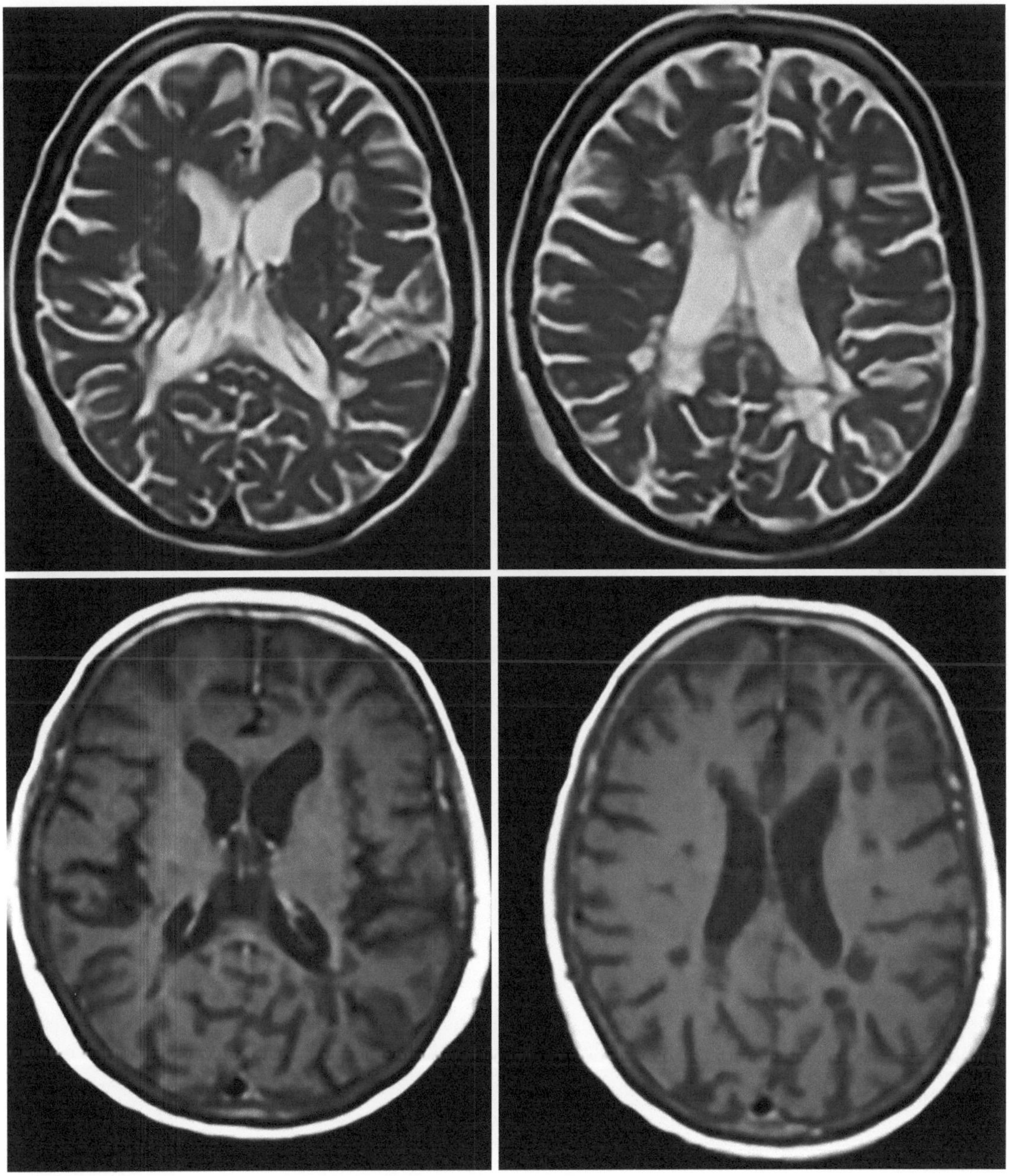

**Fig. 3** MRI images after treatment with rituximab

**Take-Home Messages**

- MRI is the gold standard for diagnosing TMS.
- [$^{18}$F]FDG PET has limited value in the differential diagnosis of brain lesions including suspected TLDs.
- TDLs are characterized by mild or moderate [$^{18}$F]fluorodopa uptake, usually with an SUV ratio with respect to the striatum <1 and might thus be of use to support differential diagnosis with respect to neoplastic lesions.

## Suggested Readings

Reich DS, Lucchinetti CF, Calabresi PA. Multiple Sclerosis. N Engl J Med. 2018;378:169–80.

Thompson AJ, Banwell BL, Barkhof F, Carroll WM, Coetzee T, Comi G, et al. Diagnosis of multiple sclerosis: 2017 revisions of the McDonald criteria. Lancet Neurol. 2018;17:162–73.

Algahtani H, Shirah B, Alassiri A. Tumefactive demyelinating lesions: a comprehensive review. Mult Scler Relat Disord. 2017;14:72–9.

Bauckneht M, Capitanio S, Raffa S, Roccatagliata L, Pardini M, Lapucci C, et al. Molecular imaging of multiple sclerosis: from the clinical demand to novel radiotracers. EJNMMI Radiopharm Chem. 2019;4:6.

# Section IV

# PET/MRI and Challenging Cases

# Case 34: Typical AD with Discordant Biomarkers

Diego Cecchin, Annachiara Cagnin, and Mariagiulia Anglani

## Clinical Presentation

A 59-year-old female with a clinical history (4 years) of mild cognitive impairment with long-term (episodic and autobiographic) and short-term memory deficits worsened in the last 2 years. The patient also presented space and time disorientation and occasional difficulties in recognizing family members. Caregivers reported increasing apathy and depression. No hallucinations have been referred by the patient or the caregiver. Sleep was preserved. A recent neuropsychological evaluation showed a global and moderate cognitive deterioration with a multi-domains cognitive impairment (MMSE 15/30). Activities of daily living (ADL) and instrumental activities of daily living (iALD) were 6/6 and 2/8, respectively, with a tendency to overlook common daily practices (hygiene, drugs intake, cooking, etc.). Past medical history was positive for cerebellar meningioma surgically treated.

The patient has been referred to a [$^{18}$F]FDG PET/MR that showed a pattern that could be associated with a diagnosis within the Alzheimer's continuum (Fig. 1). However, a CSF analysis was negative for cerebral amyloidosis:

- Total tau: >600 (*pathologic*).
- Phosphorylated Tau: >60 (*pathologic*).
- B-Amyloid: >1000 (*normal*; cut-off level for significance <500).
- Ratio B-Amyloid (1–42)/(1–40): >0.075 (*normal*; cut-off level for significance <0.055).

Because of discordant results of clinical findings and [$^{18}$F]FDG PET vs. CSF, neurologist referred the patient to a [$^{18}$F]florbetaben PET/MRI that revealed a clear, diffused uptake of radiopharmaceutical throughout the cortical and subcortical structures (Figs. 2, 3, 4).

A diagnosis of probable AD was then achieved. At present, no known genetic mutation has been found (including APP, PSEN1, PSEN2, and other genes for non-AD dementia: CHCHD10, CHMP2B, CSF1R, CST3, FUS, GRN, HNRNPA1, MAPT, PRNP, SERPINI1, SQSTM1, TARDBP, TBK1, TREM2, TUBA4A, TYROBP, UBQLN2, VAPB, VCP).

D. Cecchin (✉)
Nuclear Medicine Unit, Department of Medicine—DIMED, University-Hospital of Padova, Padova, Italy
e-mail: diego.cecchin@unipd.it

A. Cagnin
Neurology Unit, Department of Neurosciences (DNS), University-Hospital of Padova, Padova, Italy

M. Anglani
Neuroradiology Unit, University-Hospital of Padova, Padova, Italy


A. Varrone et al. (eds.), *Clinical Nuclear Medicine in Neurology*,
https://doi.org/10.1007/978-3-030-83598-9_34

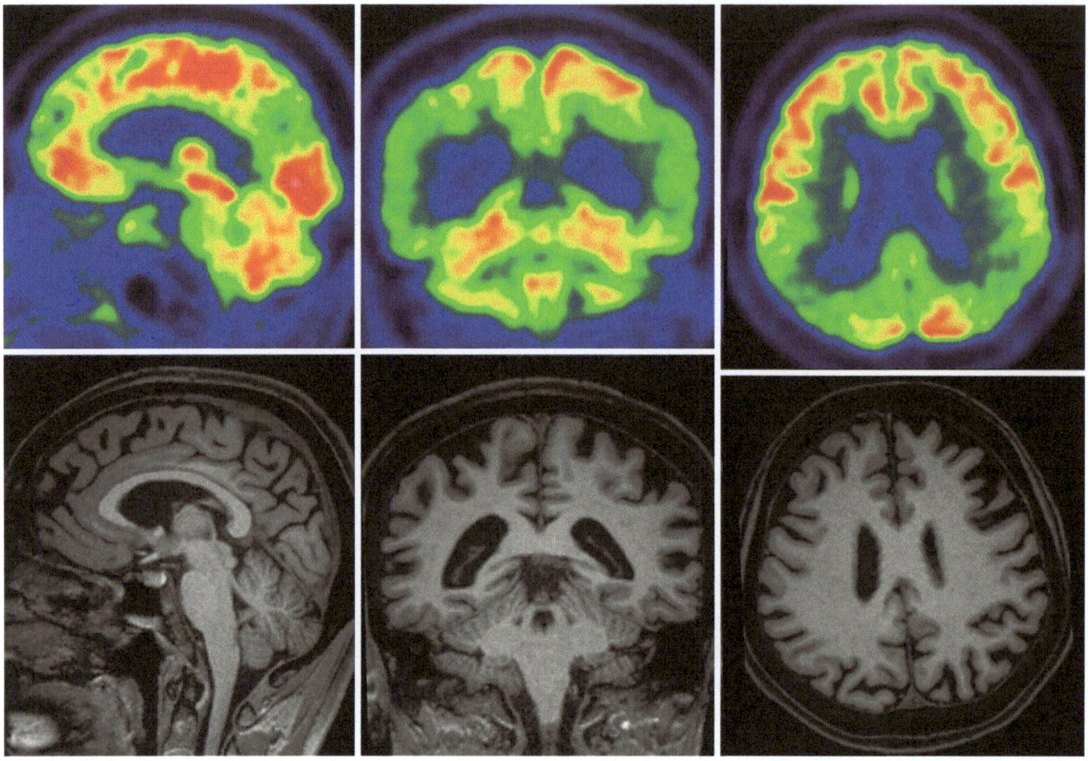

**Fig. 1** [$^{18}$F]FDG PET/MR: Sagittal (left), coronal (middle), and axial (right) [$^{18}$F]FDG (upper row) and T1 1 mm isotropic MPRAGE (lower row) showing a clear hypometabolism in parieto-temporal cortex bilaterally including precuneus and the posterior portion of the cingulate gyri. The pattern could be associated with AD pathology

## Imaging Findings

- [$^{18}$F]FDG PET/MRI (Fig. 1) showed a clear hypometabolism in parieto-temporal cortex bilaterally including precuneus and the posterior portion of the cingulate gyri. The pattern could be associated with AD continuum.
- [$^{18}$F]Florbetaben early (0–10 min after injection) amyloid scan (Fig. 3) being a "blood flow surrogate" demonstrates nearly the same pattern of [$^{18}$F]FDG (shown in Fig. 1) with the obvious exception of cerebellar perfusion.
- [$^{18}$F]Florbetaben late (90–110 min after injection) amyloid scan (Fig. 4) revealed diffuse bilateral cortical and subcortical uptake of the radiopharmaceutical. Neurodegenerative indexes were: global cortical atrophy (GCA score): 1–2; parietal atrophy (Koedam score): left: 1, right: 0; mesial temporal atrophy (MTA score): Sn: 1–2, Dx: 2; white matter lesions (Fazekas score): 1. No mesencephalic abnormalities have been reported.

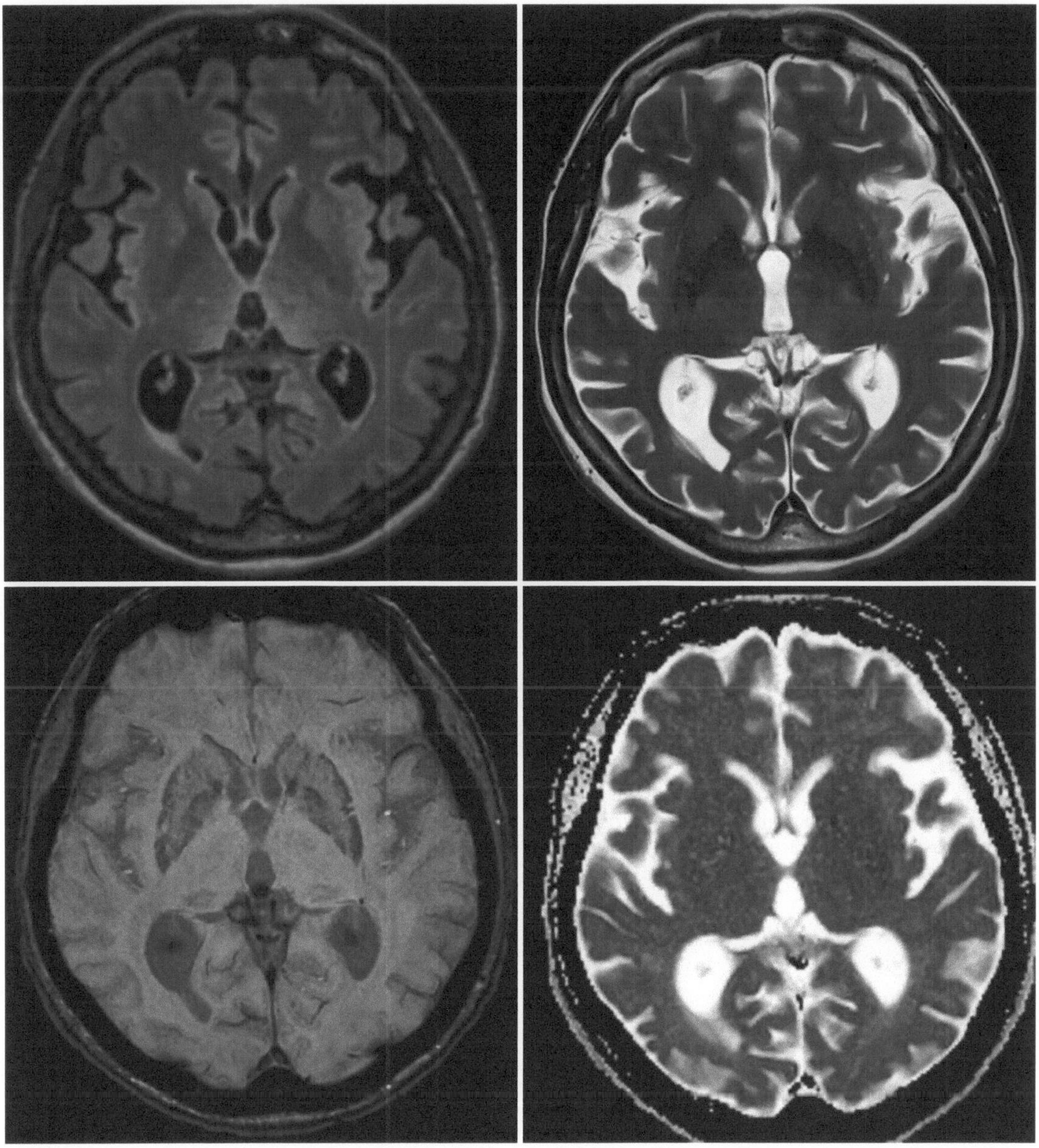

**Fig. 2** Axial T2 Flair (upper left), T2 TSE (upper right), susceptibility weighted imaging—SWI (lower left) and apparent diffusion coefficient—ADC (lower right) co-acquired to sequences in Fig. 1, demonstrating the absence of significative white matter hyperintensities, hemorrhages, and micro-bleedings

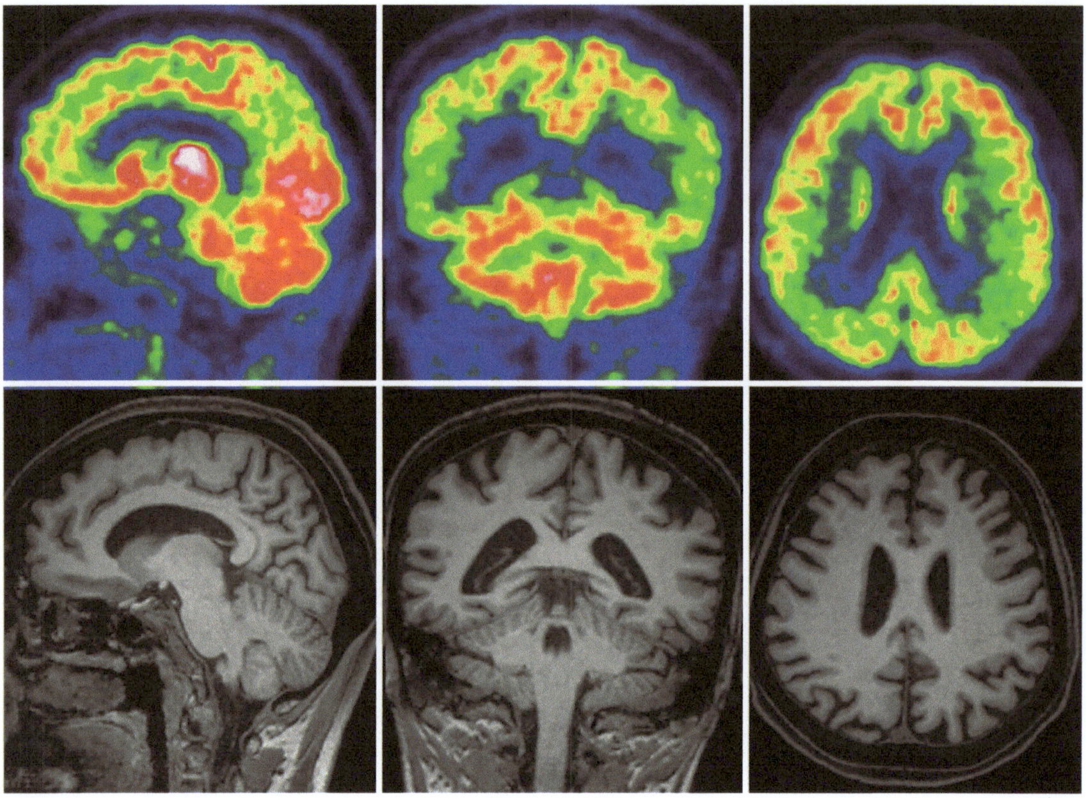

**Fig. 3** [$^{18}$F]Florbetaben PET/MR (early frame): Sagittal (left), coronal (middle), and axial (right) early (0–10 min after tracer administration) acquisition of [$^{18}$F]florbetaben (upper row) and T1 1 mm isotropic MPRAGE (lower row) that being a "blood flow surrogate" demonstrates nearly the same pattern of [$^{18}$F]FDG (shown in Fig. 1) with the obvious exception of cerebellar perfusion

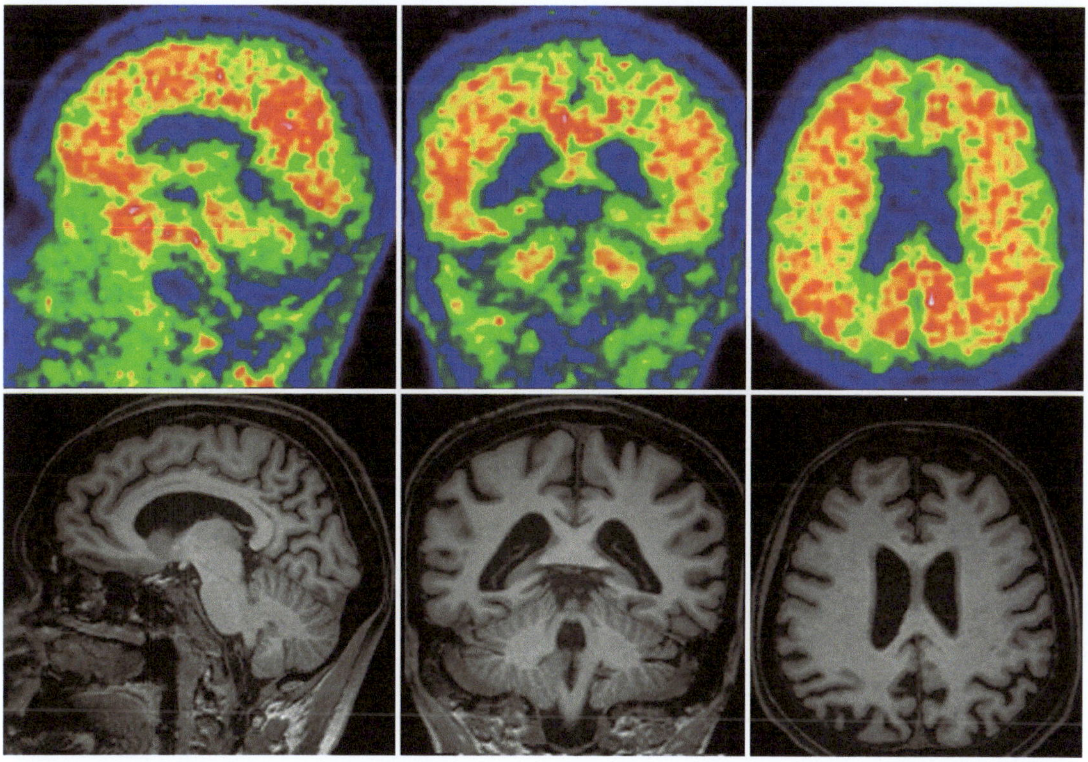

**Fig. 4** [18]F-Florbetaben PET/MR (late frame): Sagittal (left), coronal (middle), and axial (right) late (90–110 min after tracer administration) acquisition of [[18]F]florbetaben (upper row) and T1 1 mm isotropic MPRAGE (lower row), demonstrating diffuse cortical uptake of the radiopharmaceutical

**Take-Home Message**

- After a doubtful CSF study, if imaging (including [[18]F]FDG PET and MRI) and clinical findings support the diagnosis of AD, an amyloid PET could be asked to confirm or reject CSF results [1] especially in young patients (like our case) where incidental amyloidosis is less frequent.

## Reference

1. Reimand J, Groot C, Teunissen CE, Windhorst AD, Boellaard R, Barkhof F, et al. Why is amyloid-β PET requested after performing CSF biomarkers? J Alzheimers Dis. 2020;73(2):559–69. https://doi.org/10.3233/JAD-190836.

# Case 35: Frontotemporal Dementia, Behavioural Variant, Mimicker

Diego Cecchin, Annachiara Cagnin, and Mariagiulia Anglani

## Case Description

A 54-year-old male patient, obese, smoker, with a long history of arterial hypertension and sleep apnoea was referred to the emergency department for a rapid progression of lethargic state and apathetic behaviour in a few hours. In the emergency room, he performed brain CT and angio CT scans which resulted normal. The patient was then admitted to the neurological department. Assessment in the following days revealed apathic behaviour and reduced verbal fluency and severe obstructive sleep apnoea syndrome with right diaphragmatic paralysis. Repeated brain CT scan was negative. In the suspect of frontotemporal dementia and to rule out possible neoplastic conditions, the patient was referred to a whole-body and brain [$^{18}$F]FDG PET/MR (Fig. 1).

Brain [$^{18}$F]FDG PET/MR revealed a clear hypometabolism of the frontal cortex bilaterally including the anterior portion of the cingulate cortex consistent with a possible behavioural frontotemporal dementia (bvFTD). However, MR (T1-MPRAGE and T2 TSE and Flair) revealed a bilateral, anterior thalamic infarcts that could explain the frontal cortical hypometabolism due to subcortical deafferentation and the sudden onset of somnolence, apathy and executive dysfunction. Therefore, a diagnosis of bilateral strategic infarcts and resulting disconnection of the frontal cortex was established (Fig. 2).

D. Cecchin (✉)
Nuclear Medicine Unit, Department of Medicine—DIMED, University-Hospital of Padova, Padova, Italy
e-mail: diego.cecchin@unipd.it

A. Cagnin
Neurology Unit, Department of Neurosciences (DNS), University-Hospital of Padova, Padova, Italy

M. Anglani
Neuroradiology Unit, University-Hospital of Padova, Padova, Italy

## Usual Imaging Findings in Strategic Infarcts

- Single small infarct usually located in thalamus, basal ganglia (including caudate and globus pallidus), angular gyrus, and inferomedial temporal lobes.
- *MR*: T1-weighted sequences hypointense; *T1 contrast-enhanced* may enhance if acute (or early subacute); *T2/FLAIR*: hyperintense.
- *PET*: Disconnected cortical areas are usually hypometabolic using [$^{18}$F]FDG.

## Usual Clinical Presentation of Strategic Infarcts

- Strokes in left angular gyrus, left basal ganglia structures and the white matter around the left basal ganglia seem to be strategic structures


A. Varrone et al. (eds.), *Clinical Nuclear Medicine in Neurology*,
https://doi.org/10.1007/978-3-030-83598-9_35

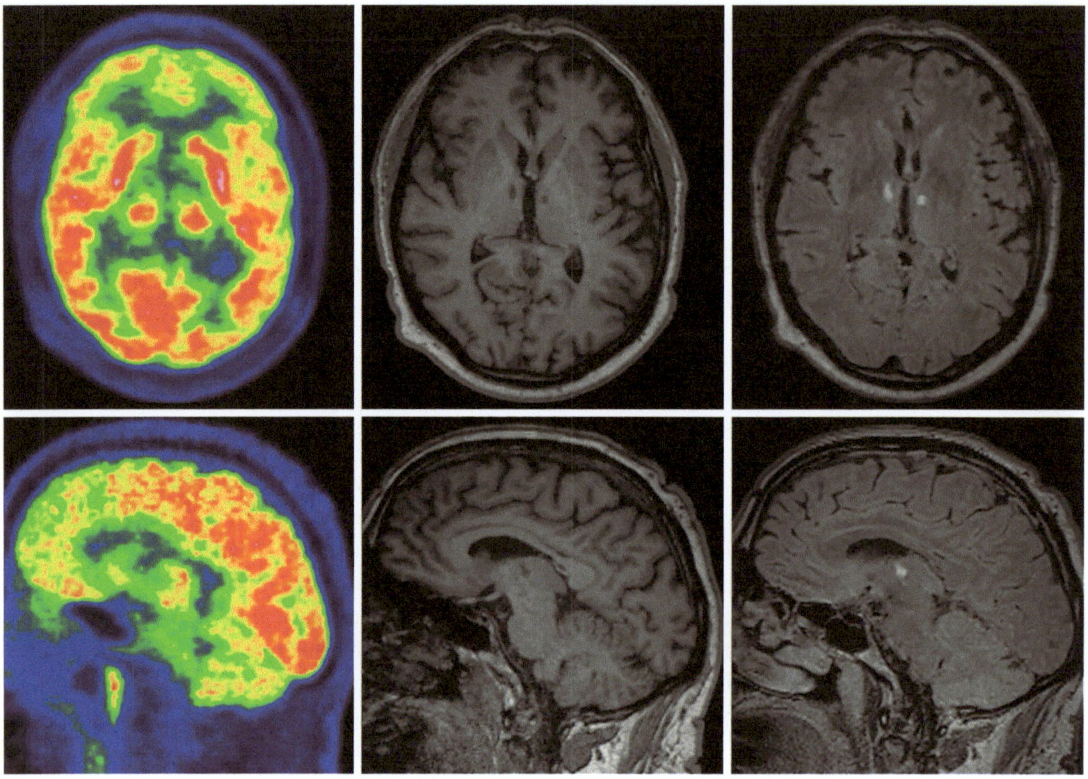

**Fig. 1** [$^{18}$F]FDG PET/MR: axial (upper row) and sagittal (lower row) [$^{18}$F]FDG (left column), T1 1 mm isotropic MPRAGE (middle column) and T2-Flair (right column) showing strategic infarcts in the anterior portion of the thalamus bilaterally (hypointense in T1 and hyperintense in T2) explaining the [$^{18}$F]FDG hypometabolism in the frontal cortex as a consequence of deafferentation (and the hypometabolism in the anterior portion of the thalamus)

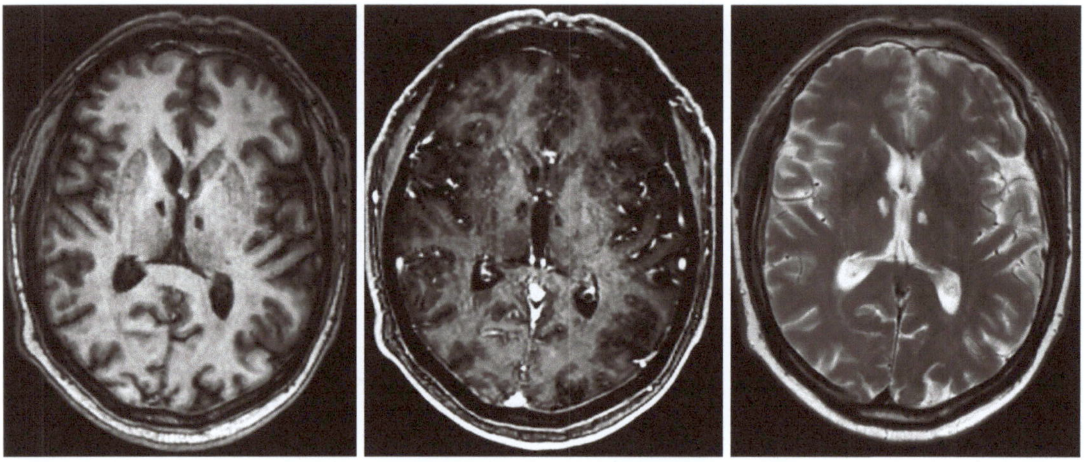

**Fig. 2** Axial T1 MPRAGE (left), contrast-enhanced T1 MPRAGE (middle), T2 TSE (right) 1 month after the acquisition of PET/MR (Fig. 1), demonstrating not significative evolution of the disease

more frequently associated with global cognitive impairment after stroke [1].

- Anterior thalamic radiation (like in our case) and forceps minor [2] seems to be involved frequently in vascular dementia; however, it seems recognized nowadays that strategic infarcts integrate into larger networks with a role in cognition. In these cases, the most mimicked neurodegenerative condition is FTD because of disconnection of the frontal cortex.

**Take-Home Message**

- Sudden clinical neurological symptoms in a young comorbid patient suggest a cerebrovascular cause. When reading a brain PET study, it is mandatory to evaluate a recent (or co-acquired) MR acquired with T1- and T2-weighted sequences to exclude possible regions of strategic infarcts that could explain symptoms and hypometabolism (and lately also loss of grey and white matter in disconnected areas).

## References


1. Lei Zhao J, Biesbroek M, Shi L, Liu W, Kuijf HJ, Chu WW, et al. Strategic infarct location for post-stroke cognitive impairment: a multivariate lesion-symptom mapping study. J Cereb Blood Flow Metab. 2018;38(8):1299–311.
2. Duering M, Zieren N, Hervé D, Jouvent E, Reyes S, Peters N, et al. Strategic role of frontal white matter tracts in vascular cognitive impairment: a voxel-based lesion-symptom mapping study in CADASIL. Brain. 2011;134:2366–75.

# Case 36: Creutzfeldt–Jakob Disease

Diego Cecchin, Carlo Gabelli, and Mariagiulia Anglani

## Clinical Presentation

A 76-year-old obese male presented at the neurology department for cognitive decline, mainly with deficits in the verbal domain (anomia and verbal perseverations). There were memory deficits and irritability. The patient showed also drowsiness, mild camptocormic posture with left arm bradykinesia, and recurrent falls. No visual disturbances or rapid eye movement sleep behavior disorders (RBD) were present. A tendency toward social isolation was also reported by the caregiver.

A neuropsychological evaluation showed an initial multi-domain deterioration (MMSE 24/30) mainly focused on the verbal domain. Activities of daily living (ADL) and instrumental activities of daily living (IALD) were 5/6 and 3/5, respectively. Because of an obstructive sleep apnea syndrome (OSAS) a continuous positive airway pressure (CPAP) during sleep was prescribed (not well tolerated).

An MR performed previously showed dilated sylvian cisterns and loss of hippocampal height bilaterally (DWI was not performed). EEG was not informative.

CSF examination showed a low concentration of amyloid beta 1–42 (383 ng/L), abnormal high total tau (1112 ng/L), and reduced 181-phosphorylated tau (40 ng/L). Amyoid-beta 1–42/P-tau ratio was normal.

In the clinical suspect of a primary progressive aphasia with parkinsonism, the patient was referred to a [$^{18}$F]FDG PET/MR.

## Imaging Findings

- [$^{18}$F]FDG PET/MR (Siemens, Erlangen, Germany) showed (Fig. 1 last column on the right) moderate cortical hypometabolism in the left temporal pole extending to the homolateral insular region. A slight hypometabolism was also observed in the mesial frontal cortex bilaterally including the anterior portion of the gyrus cinguli.
- Neurodegenerative indexes were: global cortical atrophy (GCA score): 1; parietal atrophy (Koedam score): left: 0, right: 0; mesial temporal atrophy (MTA score): Sn: 2, Dx: 2; white matter lesions (Fazekas score): 2. No

D. Cecchin (✉)
Nuclear Medicine Unit, Department of Medicine—DIMED, University-Hospital of Padova, Padova, Italy
e-mail: diego.cecchin@unipd.it

C. Gabelli
CRIC - Centro Regionale per lo Studio e la Cura dell'Invecchiamento Cerebrale, Azienda Ospedaliera di Padova, Padova, Italy
e-mail: carlo.gabelli@aopd.veneto.it

M. Anglani
Neuroradiology Unit, University-Hospital of Padova, Padova, Italy


A. Varrone et al. (eds.), *Clinical Nuclear Medicine in Neurology*,
https://doi.org/10.1007/978-3-030-83598-9_36

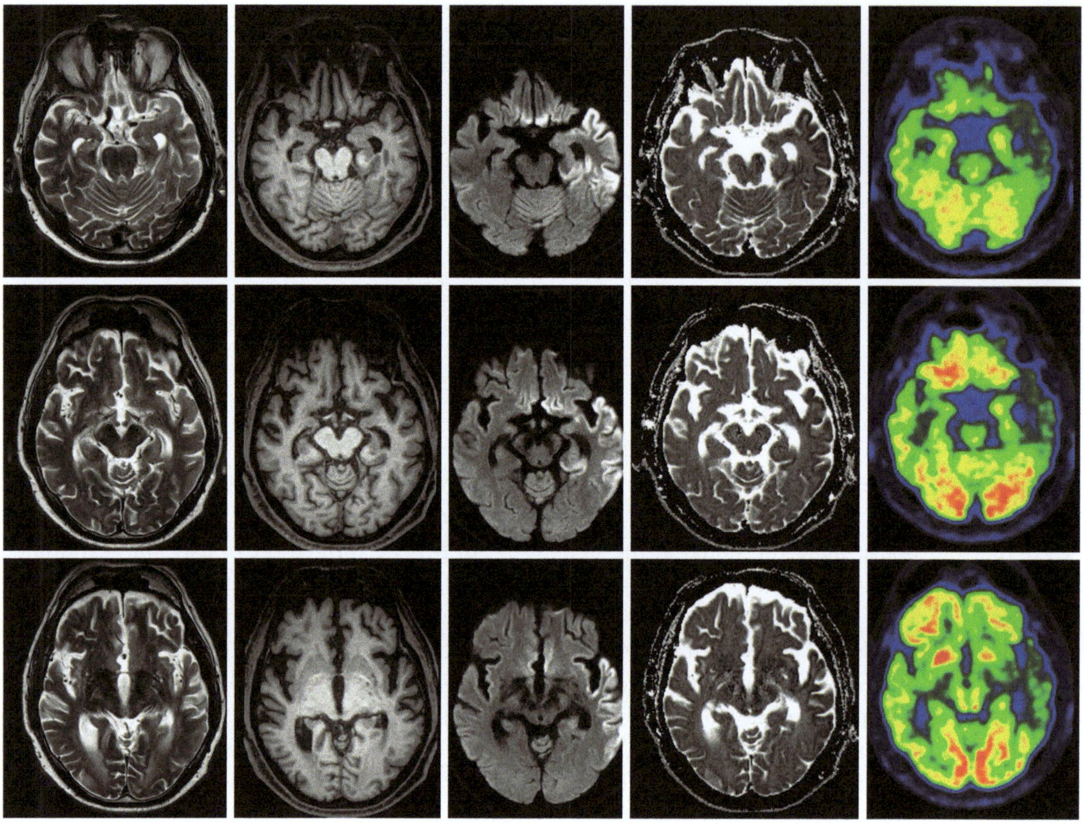

**Fig. 1** [$^{18}$F]FDG PET/MR: axial slices showing T2 TSE (first column from the left), T1 1 mm isotropic MPRAGE (second column from the left), DWI b1000 (third column from the left), ADC map (fourth column from the left), and [$^{18}$F]FDG PET (last column)

mesencephalic abnormalities have been reported.

- A high-resolution diffusion-weighted imaging (DWI) sequence (Resolve, Siemens), acquired during PET/MR, showed (using a b value of 1000 s/mm$^2$) linear hyperintensity (and hypointensity in apparent diffusion coefficient—ADC map) following the cortical rim corresponding to the [$^{18}$F]FDG hypometabolism.

An atypical (95% of cases shows hyperintensities in insula, cingulate giri, frontal cortex, and deep gray matter [1]) Creutzfeldt–Jacob disease (CJD) was supposed on the basis of DWI and PET findings.

A real-time quaking-induced conversion (RT-QuIC) assay in the CSF confirmed the diagnosis of sporadic CJD. The patient died within 6 months from the first evaluation.

**Take-Home Message**

- In protocols for neurodegenerative diseases in MR and PET/MR, a DWI sequence (ideally using high-resolution sequences) should be included to reveal linear cortical hyperintensities typical of CJD.
- Also when clinical and [$^{18}$F]FDG PET findings point to another diagnosis (like primary progressive aphasia in our case), it is useful to exclude the presence of DWI hyperintensities.
- CJD could present in an atypical form (like the temporal pole location in our case) and could increase in extent and intensity with duration [2].

## References


1. Tschampa HJ, Kallenberg K, Kretzschmar HA, et al. Pattern of cortical changes in sporadic Creutzfeldt-Jakob disease. AJNR Am J Neuroradiol. 2007;28:1114–8.
2. Eisenmenger L, Porter M-C, Carswell C, et al. Evolution of diffusion-weighted magnetic resonance imaging signal abnormality in sporadic Creutzfeldt-Jakob disease, with histopathological correlation. JAMA Neurol. 2016;73(1):76–84.

# Case 37: Atypical Upper Motor Neuron Disease

Diego Cecchin, Gianni Sorarù, and Mariagiulia Anglani

## Background

Amyotrophic lateral sclerosis (ALS)-plus refers to motor neuron disease cases with atypical features including cerebellar, extrapyramidal, or autonomic signs [1].

## Clinical Presentation

A 67-year-old man came for evaluation of progressive weakness in his left arm. He had no family history of neuromuscular diseases.

On admission, walking was ataxic with the left arm held adduct and semi-flexed; commuting of upper limbs was reduced with marked and widespread bradykinesia. Retropulsion was prominent. Pull test was positive. Passive motility was reduced at both the upper limbs due to bilateral "frozen shoulder." The examination of muscle tone showed an extrapyramidal hypertonus at elbow level, and a pyramidal hypertonus at lower limbs; there was atrophy of the left gastrocnemius muscle and quadriceps femoris. There was full paresis of the left upper limb; reflexes were 3 of 4 in the arms and legs, greater on the left side than the right side, with bilateral Hoffman sign and crossed adduction. Glabellar and palmomental reflex was present.

Hematological, immunological profile and the detection of antibodies against neuronal antigens were normal.

Neuropsychological examination revealed a dysexecutive syndrome with a mild perseveration in thoughts, behaviors, and actions, and mild impairment of working memory and short-term memory.

## Imaging and Biopsy Findings

During the admission, the patient underwent a left quadriceps muscle biopsy that showed a pattern of neurogenic atrophy in early stages.

SPET with [$^{123}$I]Ioflupane (performed to exclude nigrostriatal degeneration that could, at least partially, explain clinical presentation) did not reveal any substantial reduction of uptake of the basal ganglia.

In order to evaluate if the clinical picture could be included in a form of tauopathy, the patient underwent a brain [$^{18}$F]FDG PET-MRI (Fig. 1).

D. Cecchin (✉)
Nuclear Medicine Unit, Department of Medicine—DIMED, University-Hospital of Padova, Padova, Italy
e-mail: diego.cecchin@unipd.it

G. Sorarù
Neurology Unit, Department of Neurosciences (DNS), University-Hospital of Padova, Padova, Italy

M. Anglani
Neuroradiology Unit, University-Hospital of Padova, Padova, Italy



A. Varrone et al. (eds.), *Clinical Nuclear Medicine in Neurology*,
https://doi.org/10.1007/978-3-030-83598-9_37

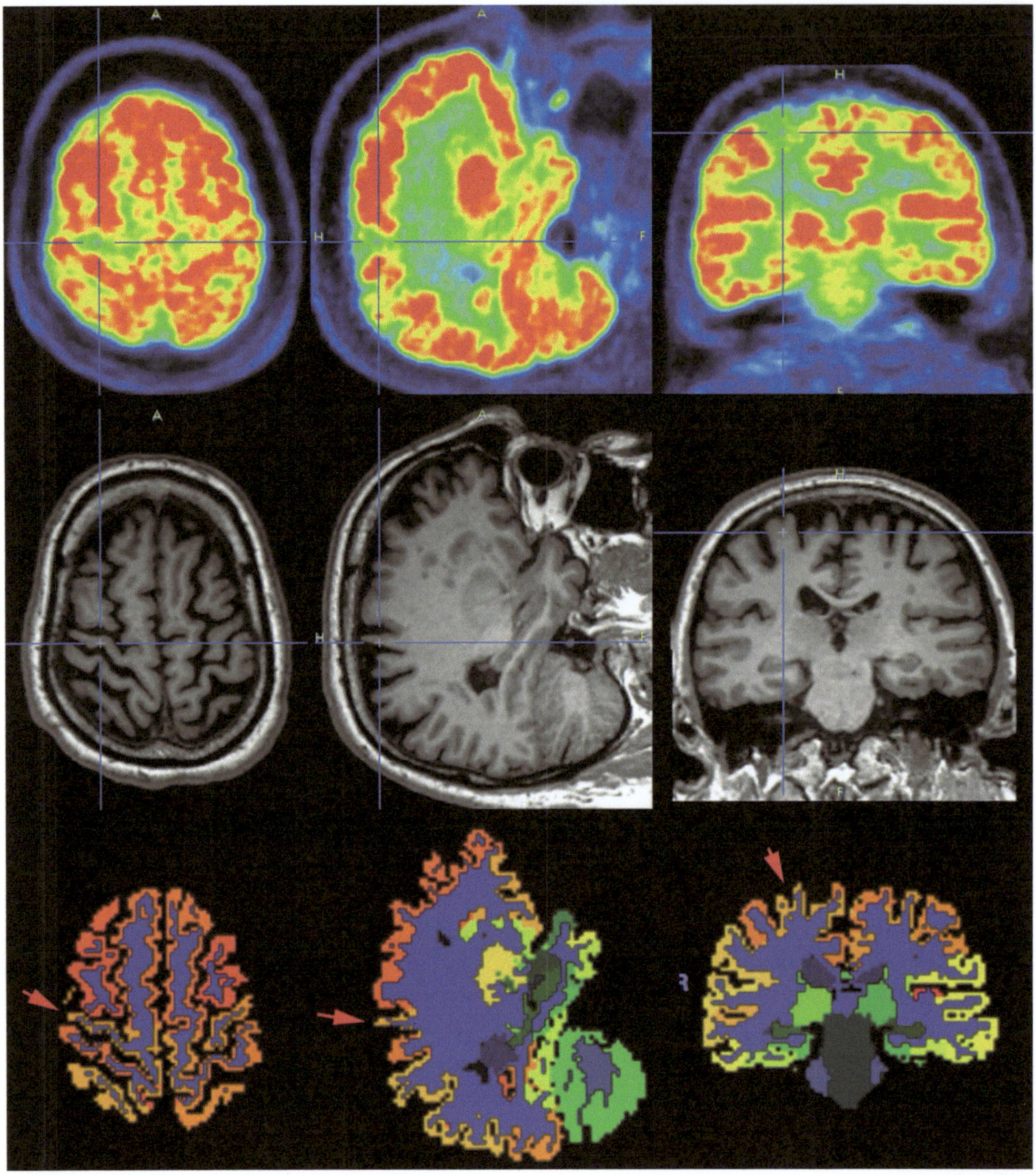

**Fig. 1** [$^{18}$F]FDG PET/MRI showing hypometabolism clearly localized at the right precentral gyrus. In the first row axial, sagittal, and coronal [$^{18}$F]FDG PET images. In the second row corresponding T1-MPRAGE images. In the third row [$^{18}$F]FDG PET corrected for partial volume effect (PVC) using MR. Red arrow shows the hypometabolic cortex on the right side

While multiple areas of an altered signal at the subcortical and periventricular white matter level were detected on FLAIR sequence, PET-MRI highlights the presence of a moderate hypometabolism localized at the right precentral gyrus, suggesting a selective degeneration of neurons of the primary motor area.

A diagnosis of amyotrophic lateral sclerosis with additional features, consistent with ALS-plus syndrome, was done.

## Discussion

Although structural T1-weighted MRI enables analysis of focal brain atrophy, in patients with ALS or ALS-plus syndrome, conventional MRI is frequently not informative, and its diagnostic use is restricted to exclusion of other mimic disorders [1, 2]. Cross-sectional voxel-based morphometry studies have yielded inconsistent results regarding the presence of atrophy in the primary motor cortex or premotor cortex in ALS and the extent of extra-motor atrophy.

[$^{18}$F]FDG-PET might represent a potential diagnostic biomarker of ALS. Widespread decreased glucose metabolism in the cerebral cortex and basal ganglia has been associated with disease duration, muscular weakness, and poor performance on the word fluency test. Conversely, hypermetabolism was noted in the midbrain [3] and medial temporal cortex of patients with ALS, particularly in patients with spinal onset. Hypermetabolism was possibly related to the reactive astrocytosis that surrounds the affected motor neurons, the descending white matter tracts fanning out from the primary motor cortex, and the brainstem.

**Take-Home Message**
PET/MRI scan with [$^{18}$F]FDG could improve diagnostic accuracy in ALS, enabling a better working definition of anatomical and functional aspects of the pathological process.

## References

1. Brooks BR, Miller RG, Swash M, Munsat TL. El Escorial revisited: revised criteria for the diagnosis of amyotrophic lateral sclerosis. Amyotroph Lateral Scler. 2000;1(5):293.
2. Turner MR, Hardiman O, Benatar M, et al. Controversies and priorities in amyotrophic lateral sclerosis. Lancet Neurol. 2013;12:310–22.
3. Cistaro A, Valentini MC, Chiò A, et al. Brain hypermetabolism in amyotrophic lateral sclerosis: a FDG PET study in ALS of spinal and bulbar onset. Eur J Nucl Med Mol Imaging. 2012;39(2):251–9.

# Case 38: Non-Lesional Epilepsy: A Tricky Case

Tatjana Traub-Weidinger, Gregor Kasprian, Christian Dorfer, Ellen Gelpi, and Ekaterina Pataraia

## Introduction

Epilepsy has a prevalence of 0.6% of the population in industrialized countries. Over 2/3 of epilepsy patients suffer from focal forms. Standard therapy using anticonvulsive drugs is however inefficient in about 30% of these patients and treatment alternatives such as surgery with the goal of a complete resection or disconnection of the epileptogenic zone are needed [1]. Surgical interventions are planned based on a variety of diagnostic tests, including functional testing and neuroimaging techniques [2]. The results of epilepsy surgery are very promising with high chance of cure, especially in temporal lobe epilepsy with significant higher seizure freedom compared to medical treatment [3]. In contrast, the localization of the seizure onset zone in non-lesional epilepsy is difficult, and the identification of epileptogenic zones, including definition of its boundaries, often remains challenging [4].

## Clinical History

We are presenting the case of a 24-year-old right-handed man. Family history in regard of seizure disorders or any other neurological diseases was negative. History of pregnancy was unremarkable, after vacuum extraction delivery, there were no further complications. The patient had febrile seizures at the age of 1 year, the further development was unremarkable, with no history of traumatic brain injury, meningitis, or encephalitis.

Seizures started at the age of 8 years. Presumably they were bilateral tonic-clonic. Treatment with oxcarbazepine was started, and

T. Traub-Weidinger (✉)
Division of Nuclear Medicine, Department of Biomedical Imaging and Image-Guided Therapy, Medical University of Vienna, Vienna, Austria
e-mail: tatjana.traub-weidinger@meduniwien.ac.at

G. Kasprian
Division of Neuro- and Musculoskeletal Radiology, Department of Biomedical Imaging and Image-Guided Therapy, Medical University of Vienna, Vienna, Austria

C. Dorfer
Department of Neurosurgery, Medical University of Vienna, Vienna, Austria

E. Gelpi
Division of Neuropathology and Neurochemistry, Department of Neurology, Medical University of Vienna, Medical University of Vienna, Vienna, Austria

E. Pataraia
Department of Neurology, Medical University of Vienna, Vienna, Austria



A. Varrone et al. (eds.), *Clinical Nuclear Medicine in Neurology*,
https://doi.org/10.1007/978-3-030-83598-9_38

since the seizures continued, it was switched to valproic acid. During the subsequent 3 years, he was seizure-free, the antiepileptic medication was tapered and ultimately stopped, and the patient stayed seizure-free for 4 years without any medication. At the age of 15 years, the seizures re-appeared and treatment with oxcarbazepine was reinitialized. Since seizure-freedom was not achieved, antiepileptic medication was changed several times including oxcarbazepine, valproic acid, lamotrigine, levetiracetam, perampanel, and lacosamide in different combinations. The seizure frequency was 2 times a week. The patient described an epigastric aura and a sensation of thirst at the beginning of seizure, followed by consciousness impairment. His family described frequent swallowing; very seldom did the patient have a generalized tonic-clonic seizure. Finally, at the age of 23 years, he was referred to a tertiary epilepsy center.

## Presurgical Work-Up

### Prolonged Video-EEG Monitoring

Video-EEG monitoring with scalp electrodes according to 10–20 International System with additional anterior temporal electrodes and bilaterally placed sphenoidal electrodes was performed for 5 days. Six seizures were registered after tapering of medication. All seizures started with an epigastric aura followed by a sensation of thirst/ictal drinking, impaired awareness and oral automatisms. No bilateral tonic-clonic seizures were documented during video-EEG monitoring. Ictal EEG showed rhythmic theta activity in the right mesial temporal area (Sp2) in all seizures (see Fig. 1). There were only few spikes registered on the right side in the mesial temporal area (Sp2) during the interictal EEG (see Fig. 2).

### Neuropsychological Testing

The preoperative neuropsychological testing showed an almost unaffected neuropsychological profile.

### Structural and Functional MRI

High-resolution MRI applying the epilepsy protocol as recommended by the International League against Epilepsy (ILAE) [5] showed an abnormal gyral configuration at the transition of the right inferior frontal gyrus and the insula with the suspicion of a discrete cortical thickening. There were no associated T1-weighted or T2-weighted/FLAIR signal alterations in this region. Still, a very subtle locally circumscribed focal cortical dysplasia was suspected. No other obvious lesions were detected by serial MR examinations. In the functional MRI language, functions were lateralized to the left hemisphere.

### 2-[$^{18}$F]Fluoro-2-Deoxy-D-Glucose (FDG) PET/MR

As recently established, the patient was further examined with an epilepsy imaging protocol combining nuclear medicine and radiology procedures of a fully integrated PET/MR combined system. This protocol allows to noninvasively estimate the regional absolute metabolic rate of glucose (MRGlc in μmol/100 g/min) in addition to a visual analysis of PET and MRI [6, 7]. There was no FDG hypometabolic area correlating to the right inferior frontal gyrus or right anterior insula as described as a structural abnormality by MRI, which corresponded well with the EEG results (see Fig. 3). Moreover, PET imaging revealed a reduced tracer uptake in the right anterior temporal lobe (see Fig. 4). Additional

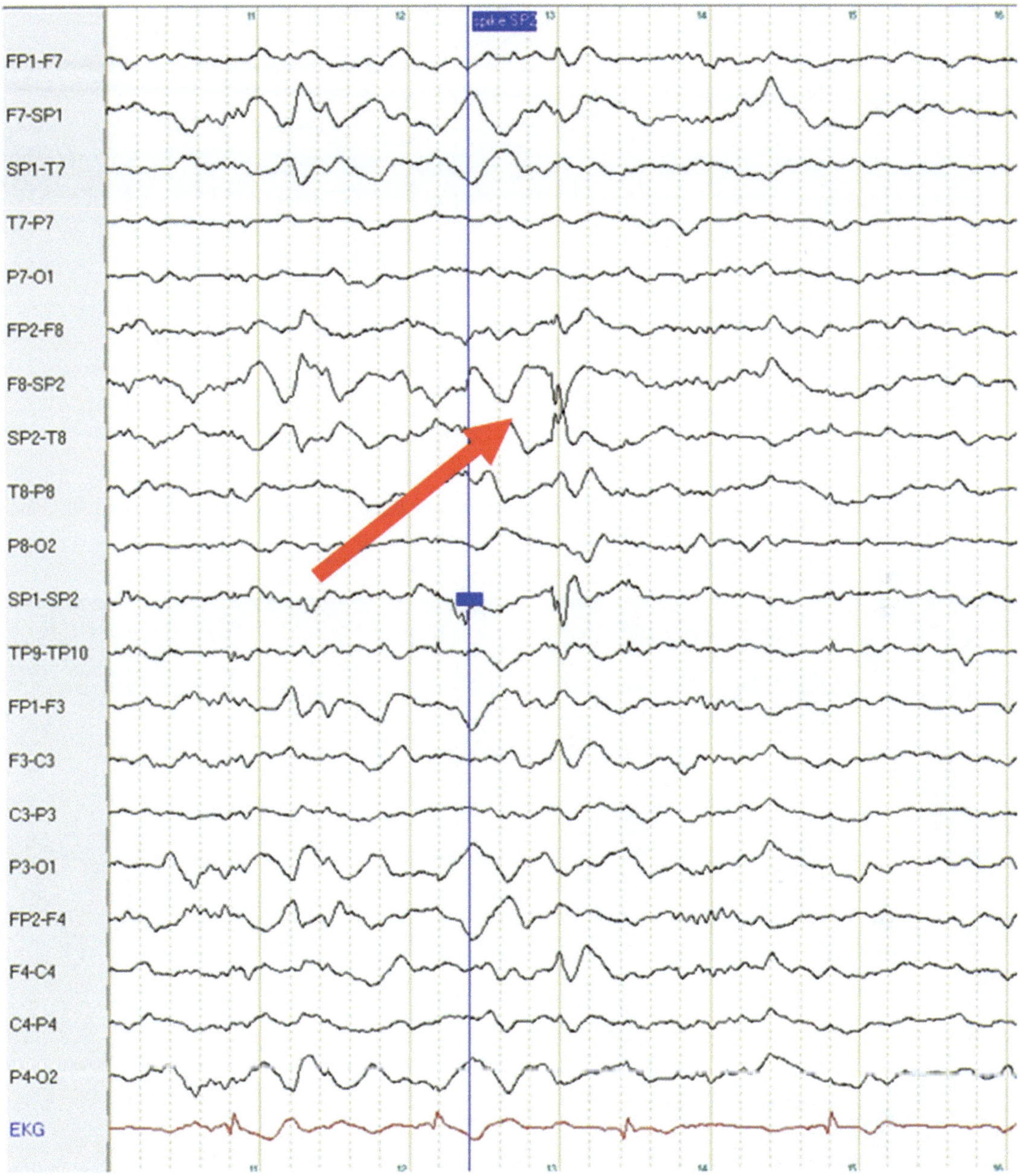


**Fig. 1** Ictal scalp EEG; Longitudinal bipolar montage with additional sphenoidal electrodes, 30 mm/s, 70 mV. Ictal EEG pattern, rhythmic theta activity right temporal (red arrow)

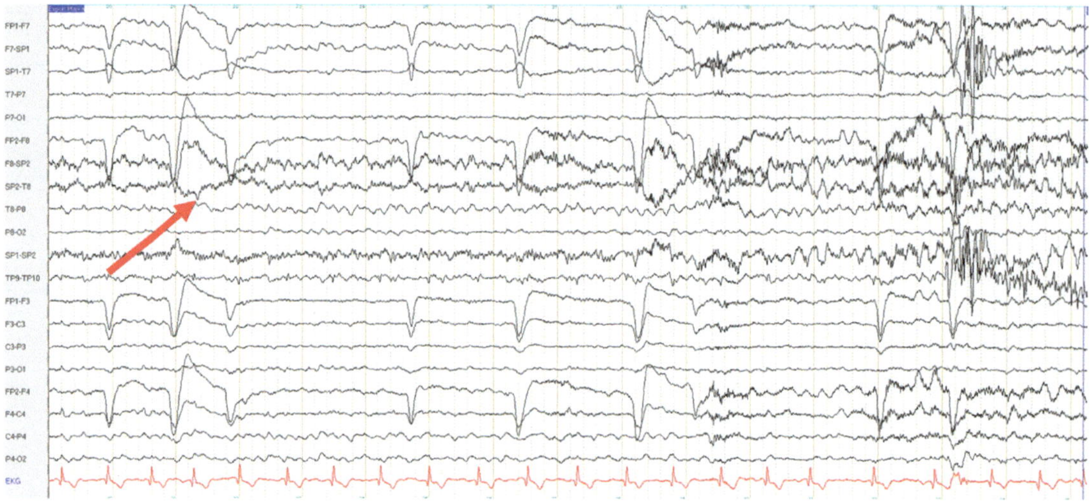


**Fig. 2** Interictal scalp EEG; Longitudinal bipolar montage with additional sphenoidal electrodes, 30 mm/s, 70 mV. Interictal spike right mesial temporal, electrode SP2 (red arrow)

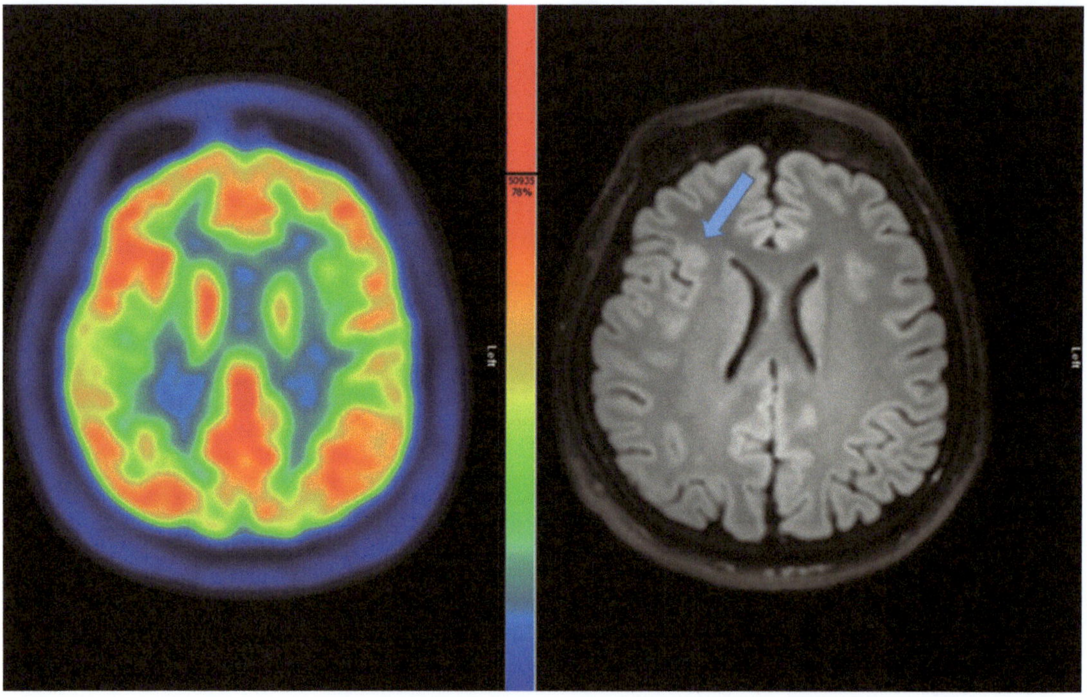


**Fig. 3** FDG PET/MR. Axial FDG PET (left side) and corresponding Flair MRI sequence (right side) showing a very subtle local thickening of the right inferior frontal gyrus (arrow) leading to the suspicion of a type 1 focal cortical dysplasia. No FDG hypometabolism nor EEG abnormality was found in this region at the interface between of the right gyrus frontalis interior and the insula

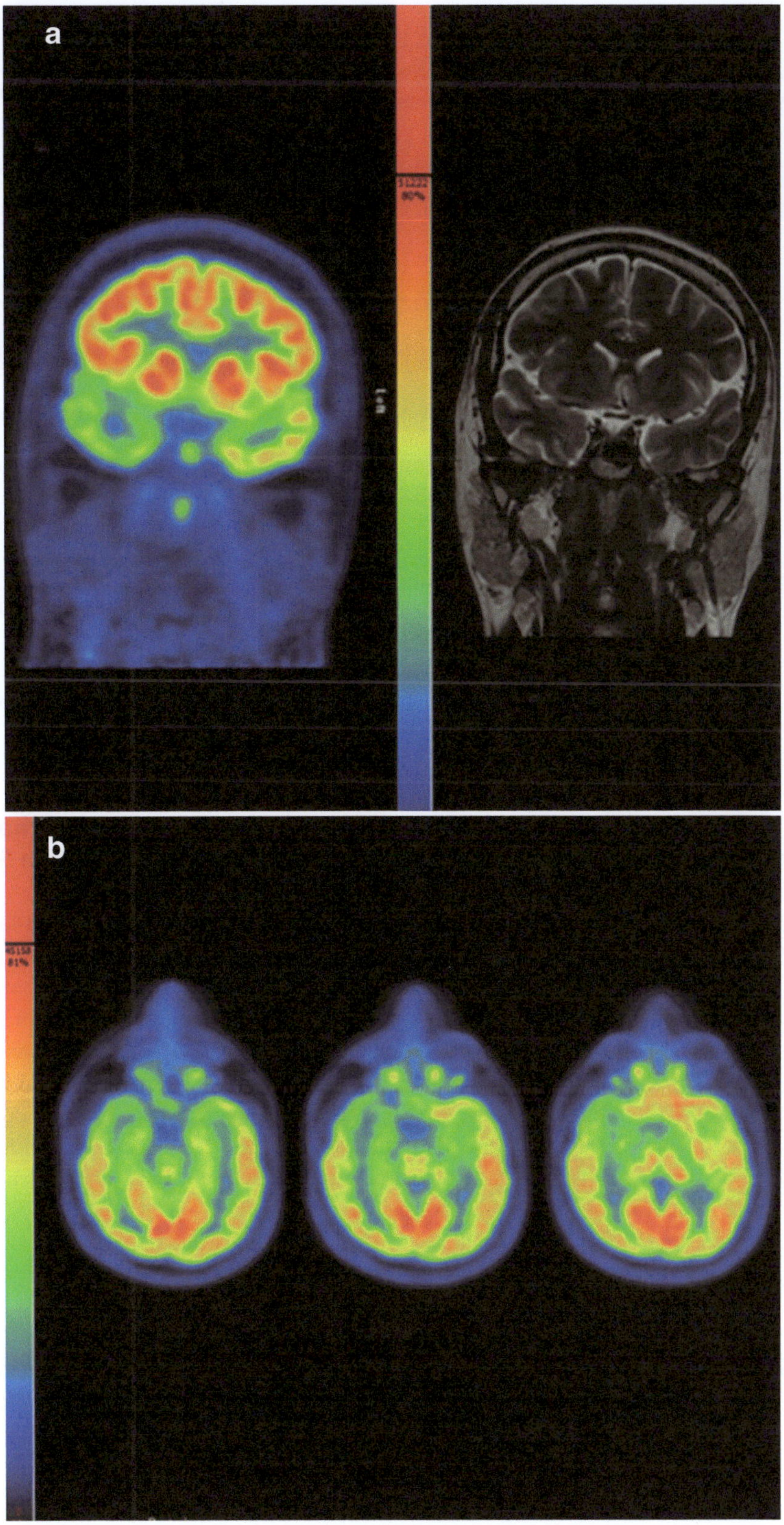


**Fig. 4** (**a**, **b**) FDG PET/MR imaging. Coronal (**a**) and axial views (**b**) of FDG PET with reduced tracer uptake in the right ventral temporal lobe corresponding to MRI Flair sequence without any structural abnormality. The hypometabolic area included the lateral, polar, and mesial part of the right anterior temporal lobe

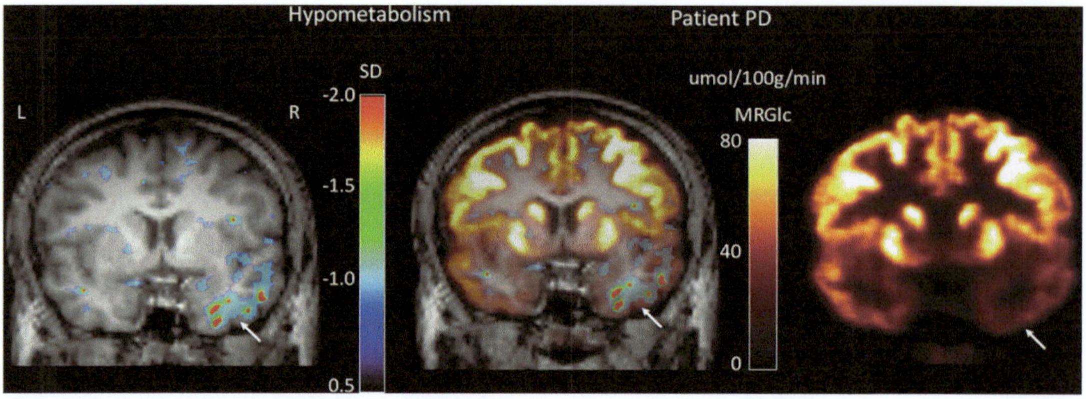


**Fig. 5** Absolute FDG quantification results based on an indirect arterial input function developed method recorded during the PET/MR examination. The abnormality map overlaid onto the patient's structural MR scan shows a significant focal hypometabolic area [> 2 standard deviations (SD) of control mean] in the right temporal lobe (white arrow). The color scale represents the SD below normal mean MRGlc at the location of each individual voxel (*left*). Overlay of the abnormality map onto the MRGlc and structural MR images (*center*). Focally decreased MRGlc area in the right temporal lobe (*right*)

calculation of the noninvasive absolute metabolic rate of glucose confirmed the visual analysis and revealed the maximal reduction of MRGlc in the basal and mesial areas of the right anterior temporal lobe (see Fig. 5). No further abnormalities were found in the right frontal lobe.

## Invasive Video-EEG Monitoring

Based on the results of video-EEG monitoring (clinical semiology, ictal, and interictal EEG), MRI, neuropsychological testing, and 18F-FDG-PET, a non-lesional right mesial temporal epilepsy was suspected. The patient was subjected to invasive video-EEG monitoring after discussing the case at the interdisciplinary epilepsy surgery board. Depth electrodes were placed into right mesial structures (amygdala and hippocampus), in the temporal pole, in the anterior insula and in the right inferior frontal gyrus (area of suspected lesion) (see Fig. 6). During invasive recordings, four focal seizures with impaired awareness were recorded. The clinical semiology was similar to the seizures observed during scalp-EEG monitoring: the patient had epigastric aura and sensation of thirst, behavioral arrest, and oral automatisms. Ictal EEG showed seizure onset in the region of the temporal electrodes. No seizure activity was recorded in the electrodes which were placed in the MRI suspected lesion in the frontal lobe (see Fig. 7).

## Surgery, Histopathology, and Postoperative Surgical Outcome

The results of invasive EEG recordings could clearly identify the seizure onset zone in the right temporal lobe, thus confirming that the radiologically suspected lesion in the right frontal lobe was not epileptogenic. The patient underwent anteromesial temporal lobe resection with intraoperative electrocorticography. During the surgery, a small temporobasal encephalocele—which could only be retrospectively identified by MRI—was found and also removed. Histopathology of the resected tissue showed mild malformation of cortical development in the temporal pole, almost unaffected mesial structures, and hamartia with glioneural cells in the region of the resected encephalocele (see Fig. 8). Postoperatively, the patient has now been seizure-free for 8 months.

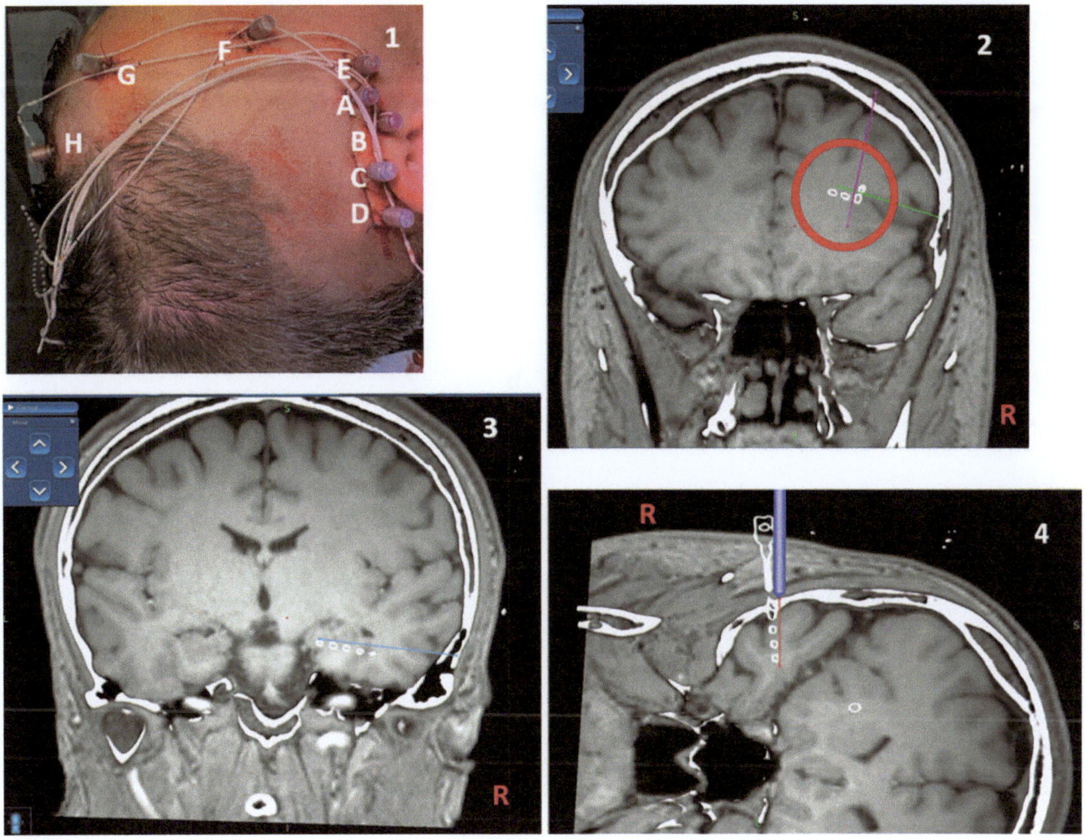


**Fig. 6** Overview of the intraoperative depth electrodes placed in the right hemisphere: (1) Depth electrodes A, B, C, and D—in mesial structures; depth electrode E—in temporal pole; depth electrodes F and G—in suspected lesion right frontal; and depth electrode H—in anterior insula. (2) Depth electrodes F and G—suspected frontal lesion (red circle). (3) Depth electrode B—mesial temporal area. (4) Depth electrode E—temporal pole

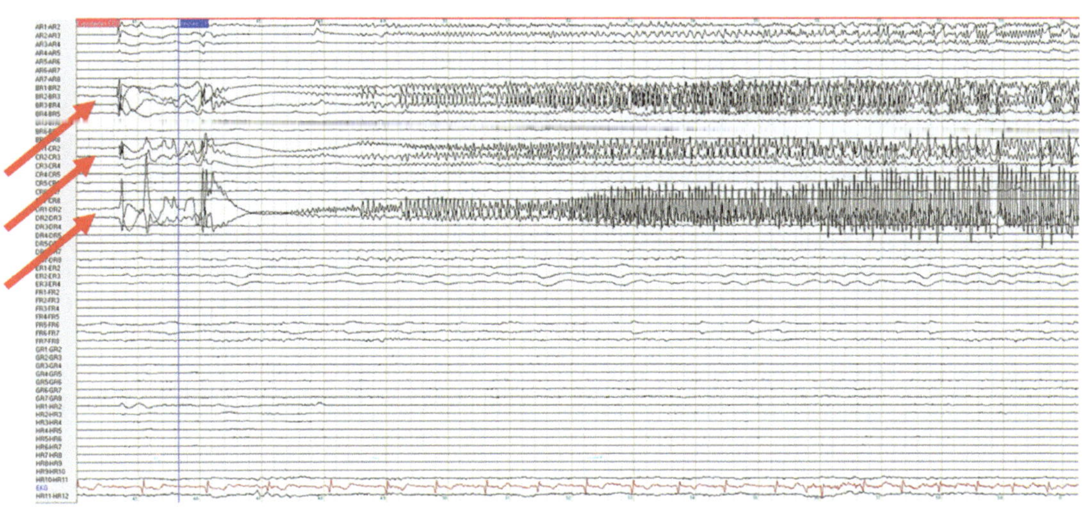

**Fig. 7** Invasive EEG, ictal EEG onset pattern, high-frequency paroxysmal activity in distal contacts of the electrodes B, C, and D, mesial temporal (red arrows)

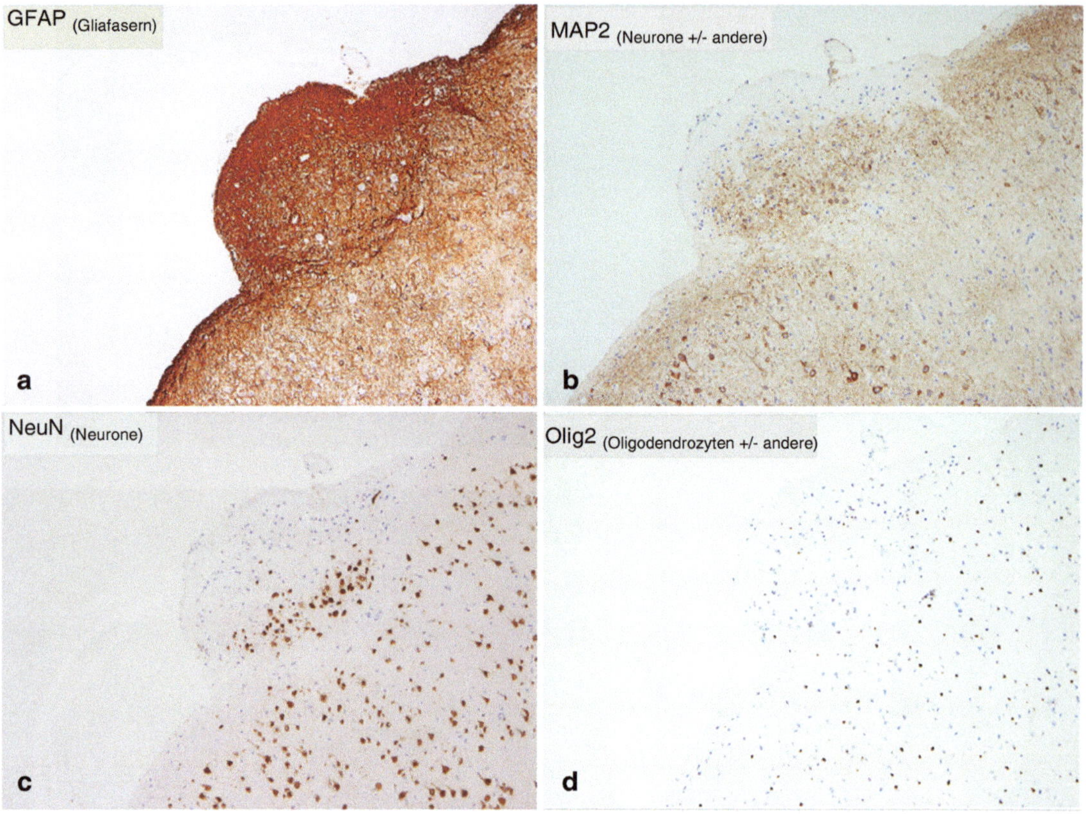


**Fig. 8** Histological examination revealed a small nodular lesion at the cortical surface protruding into the subarachnoidal space (**a**: immunohistochemistry for glial fibrillary acidic protein GFAP). (**b**, **c**) This nodule is constituted by an irregular admixture of neuronal (**b**: immunohistochemistry for microtubule-associated protein MAP 2 and **c**: for NeuN), and oligodendroglial elements (**d**: immunohistochemistry for Olig2) suggestive of a small hamartomatous lesion. In addition, GFAP shows an extensive subpial gliosis with a band-like increase of astrocytic processes along the cortical surface (**a**, **d**) and a patchy cortical gliosis (**a**). Original magnification: (**a**) ×40, (**b**–**d**) ×100

## Closing Remarks

It is well accepted that cortical hypometabolism depicted by FDG-PET provides valuable information with respect to the location of electrophysiologically confirmed seizure onset zones [8]. In non-lesional patients, FDG-PET imaging may be useful as it can lateralize and even regionalize potentially epileptogenic cortical regions to guide intracranial electrode placement and consecutively trigger surgical approach [9, 10]. However, more detailed analysis of the spatial relationship between glucose hypometabolic areas and intracranial EEG-based seizure onset zones exhibits sometimes a complex association between functional and electrophysiological data that are difficult to untangle in the absence of absolute metabolic rate of glucose (MRGlc in μmol/100 g/min) estimation [7]. In the presented case report, visual and quantitative imaging supported the clinical hypothesis for better defining the epileptogenic zone.

**Take-Home Message**

Integrated FDG PET/MRI allows structural analysis with MRI but also determination of potentially epileptogenic cortical regions in non-lesional epilepsy with FDG PET in one session. Additional non-invasive estimation of regional absolute metabolic rate of glucose has an added clinical value in the detection of more subtle hypometabolic brain areas that might be missed in clinical readings.

## References

1. Engel J Jr. Update on surgical treatment of the epilepsies. Summary of the second international palm desert conference on the surgical treatment of the epilepsies (1992). Neurology. 1993;43(8):1612–7.
2. Rosenow F, Lüders H. Presurgical evaluation of epilepsy. Brain. 2001;124(Pt 9):1683–700.
3. Engel J Jr, McDermott MP, Wiebe S, Langfitt JT, Stern JM, Dewar S, Sperling MR, Gardiner I, Erba G, Fried I, Jacobs M, Vinters HV, Mintzer S, Kieburtz K. Early Randomized Surgical Epilepsy Trial (ERSET) Study Group. Early surgical therapy for drug- resistant temporal lobe epilepsy: a randomized trial. JAMA. 2012;307:922–30.
4. Roper SN. Surgical treatment of the extratemporal epilepsies. Epilepsia. 2009;50(Suppl 8):69–74.
5. Wellmer J, Quesada CM, Rothe L, Elger CE, Bien CG, Urbach H. Proposal for a magnetic resonance imaging protocol for the detection of epileptogenic lesions at early outpatient stages. Epilepsia. 2013;54:1977–87.
6. Sundar LK, Muzik O, Rischka L, Hahn A, Rausch I, Lanzenberger R, Hienert M, Klebermass EM, Füchsel FG, Hacker M, Pilz M, Pataraia E, Traub-Weidinger T, Beyer T. Towards quantitative [18F]FDG-PET/MRI of the brain: automated MR-driven calculation of an image-derived input function for the non-invasive determination of cerebral glucose metabolic rates. J Cereb Blood Flow Metab. 2019;39(8):1516–30.
7. Traub-Weidinger T, Muzik O, Sundar LKS, Aull-Watschinger S, Beyer T, Hacker M, Hahn A, Kasprian G, Klebermass EM, Lanzenberger R, Mitterhauser M, Pilz M, Rausch I, Rischka L, Wadsak W, Pataraia E. Utility of absolute quantification in non-lesional extratemporal lobe epilepsy using FDG PET/MR imaging. Front Neurol. 2020;11:54. https://doi.org/10.3389/fneur.2020.00054.
8. Willmann O, Wennberg R, May T, Woermann FG, Pohlmann-Eden B. The contribution of 18F FDG PET in preoperative epilepsy surgery evaluation for patients with temporal lobe epilepsy: a meta-analysis. Seizure. 2007;16(6):509–20.
9. Henry TR, Sutherling WW, Engel J Jr, Risinger MW, Levesque MF, Mazziotta JC, Phelps ME. Interictal cerebral metabolism in partial epilepsies of neocortical origin. Epilepsy Res. 1991;10(2–3):174–82.
10. Salamon N, Kung J, Shaw SJ, Koo J, Koh S, Wu JY, Lerner JT, Sankar R, Shields WD, Engel J Jr, Fried I, Miyata H, Yong WH, Vinters HV, Mathern GW. FDG-PET/MRI coregistration improves detection of cortical dysplasia in patients with epilepsy. Neurology. 2008;71:1594–601.

# Case 39: Limbic Encephalitis

Diego Cecchin, Marco Zoccarato,
and Mariagiulia Anglani

## Clinical Presentation

A 65-year-old woman with a history of mild cognitive deficit (short-term memory and attention) in the last year. The patient developed recurrent confusional states, confabulation, aggressive behaviors, and delusions. Complained also episodes of epigastric aura with "feeling of strangeness." Frequent episodes of dystonic contraction of the left upper limb and hemifacial spasm were reported by the caregiver. These episodes were interpreted as faciobrachial dystonic seizures (FBDS). Therapy with levetiracetam and valproate was started with poor control of seizures.

Electroencephalography: intercritical left temporal spikes. CSF: normal cell and protein content, negative oligo-clonal bands. A brain and body [$^{18}$F]FDG PET/MR was requested in the suspect of an autoimmune encephalitis.

D. Cecchin (✉)
Nuclear Medicine Unit, Department of Medicine—DIMED, University-Hospital of Padova, Padova, Italy
e-mail: diego.cecchin@unipd.it

M. Zoccarato
Neurology Unit—OSA, University-Hospital of Padova, Padova, Italy

M. Anglani
Neuroradiology Unit, University-Hospital of Padova, Padova, Italy

Anti-neural antibody screening disclosed anti-LGI1 abs on both serum and CSF. The patient was diagnosed with limbic encephalitis according to Graus criteria (2016). Oncological screening was negative. Treatment with steroids, plasma-exchange, and lately, rituximab improved the behavioral and epileptic features, with residual mild memory deficits.

## Imaging Findings

- The first [$^{18}$F]FDG PET/MRI (Fig. 1) in the acute phase showed, in an uncooperant patient (only a 5 min scan was tolerated by the patient), a clear hypermetabolism in the amygdala bilaterally and in the striatum bilaterally as compared to the rest of the brain that showed a global cortical hypometabolism.
- The second (Fig. 2) [$^{18}$F]FDG PET/MRI (3 months after the exam showed in Fig. 1) showed a normalization of the hypermetabolism in the left amygdala and a decrease of the hypermetabolism in the right amygdala with increased uptake in the right hippocampus (corresponding to signal abnormalities in T2 FLAIR). The brain cortex (as compared to the striatum) demonstrated a nearly normalized metabolism with the exception of the occipital cortex.


A. Varrone et al. (eds.), *Clinical Nuclear Medicine in Neurology*,
https://doi.org/10.1007/978-3-030-83598-9_39

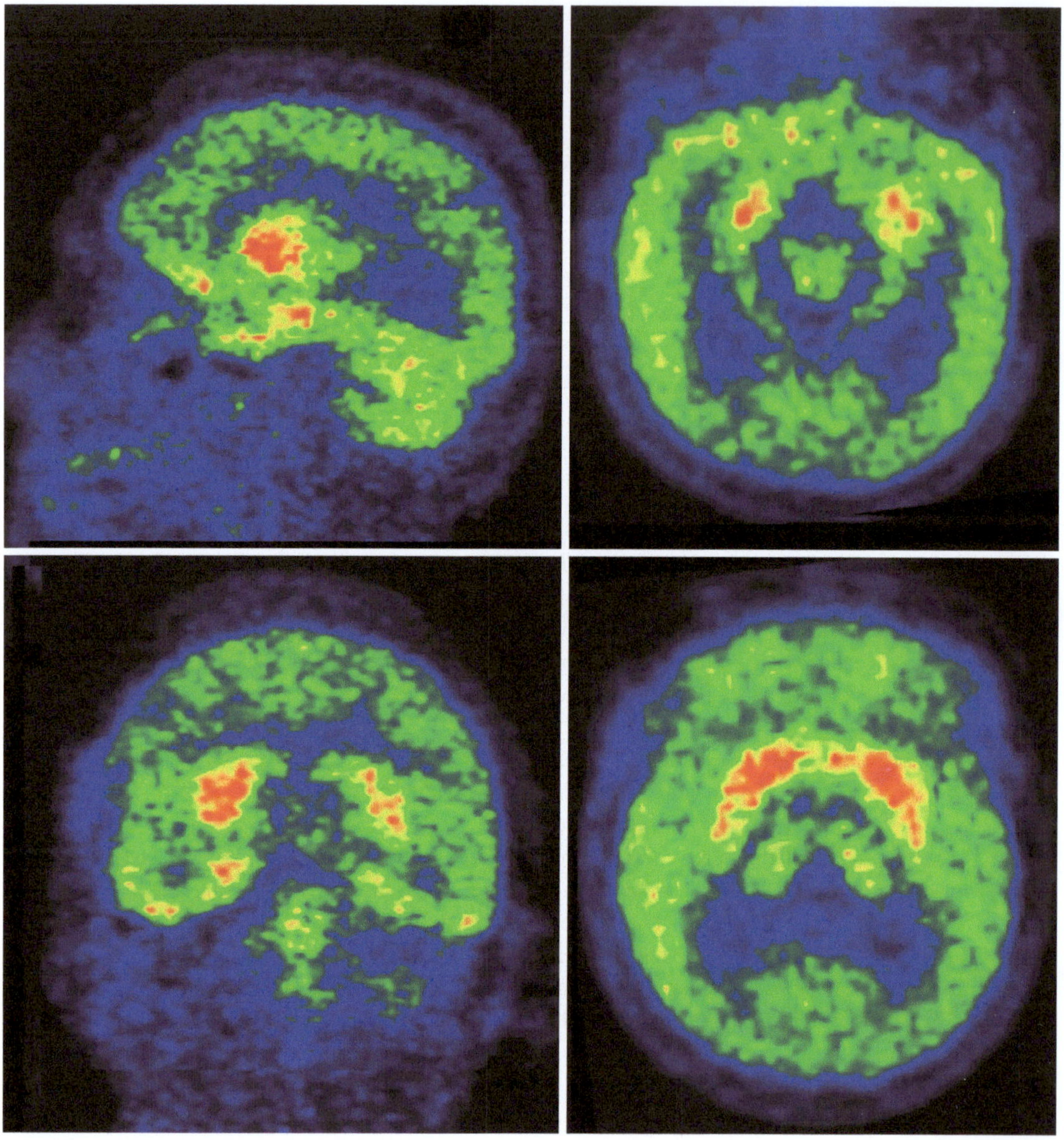

**Fig. 1** [$^{18}$F]FDG PET: sagittal (upper left), coronal (lower left), axial (upper and lower right) [$^{18}$F]FDG PET showing, in an uncooperant patient (only a 5 min scan was tolerated), a clear hypermetabolism in the amygdala bilaterally (upper right) and in the striatum bilaterally (lower right) as compared to the rest of the brain that showed a global cortical hypometabolism

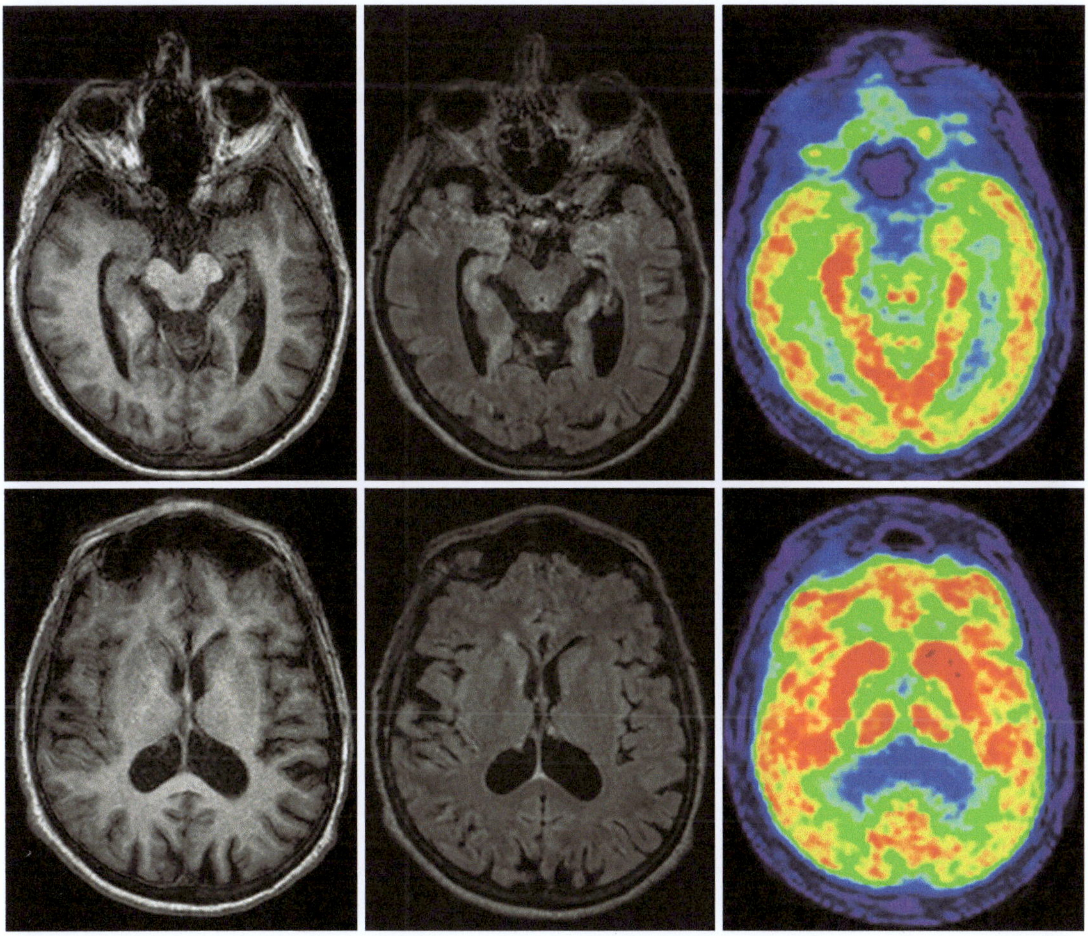

**Fig. 2** [$^{18}$F]FDG PET: axial isotropic (1 mm$^3$) T1-MPRAGE (left column), T2 Flair (middle column), [$^{18}$F]FDG PET (right column) showing (3 months after the exam showed in Fig. 1) a normalization of the hypermetabolism in the left amygdala and a decrease of the hypermetabolism in the right amygdala with increased uptake in the right hippocampus (corresponding to signal abnormalities in T2 FLAIR). The brain cortex (as compared to the striatum) demonstrated a nearly normalized metabolism with the exception of the occipital cortex

**Take-Home Message**

- FBDS are typical manifestation of LGI1 limbic encephalitis; the patient is usually unaware, and the episodes are reported by the caregiver.
- Finding of normal CSF should not exclude a diagnosis of autoimmune encephalitis.
- Metabolic imaging in limbic encephalitis with LGI1 abs can show, in addition to hypermetabolism of temporo-mesial structures (mainly hippocampus and amygdala), involvement (sometime exclusive) of basal ganglia, especially in patients with FBDS.

## Further Reading

Graus F, Titulaer MJ, Balu R, et al. A clinical approach to diagnosis of autoimmune encephalitis. Lancet Neurol. 2016;15(4):391–404.

Morbelli S, Zoccarato M, Bauckneht M, et al. 18F-FDG-PET and MRI in autoimmune encephalitis: a systematic review of brain findings. Clin Transl Imaging. 2018;6:151–68.

Shin YW, Lee ST, Shin JW, et al. VGKC-complex/LGI1-antibody encephalitis: clinical manifestations and response to immunotherapy. J Neuroimmunol. 2013;265(1–2):75–81.